A BEHAVIORAL ATLAS
OF THE RAT BRAIN

A BEHAVIORAL ATLAS OF THE RAT BRAIN

ROBERT THOMPSON

Department of Psychology
Louisiana State University
Baton Rouge, Louisiana

NEW YORK   OXFORD UNIVERSITY PRESS   1978

Copyright © by Oxford University Press, Inc. 1978

Library of Congress Cataloging in Publication Data

Thompson, Robert, 1927–
A behavioral atlas of the rat brain.
Bibliography: p.
Includes index.
1. Brain—Atlases. 2. Brain—Localization
of functions. 3. Rats—Anatomy. I. Title.
QL937.T46   599'.322   77-27089
ISBN 0-19-502268-8   ISBN 0-19-502269-6 pbk.

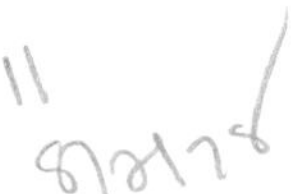

Printed in the United States of America

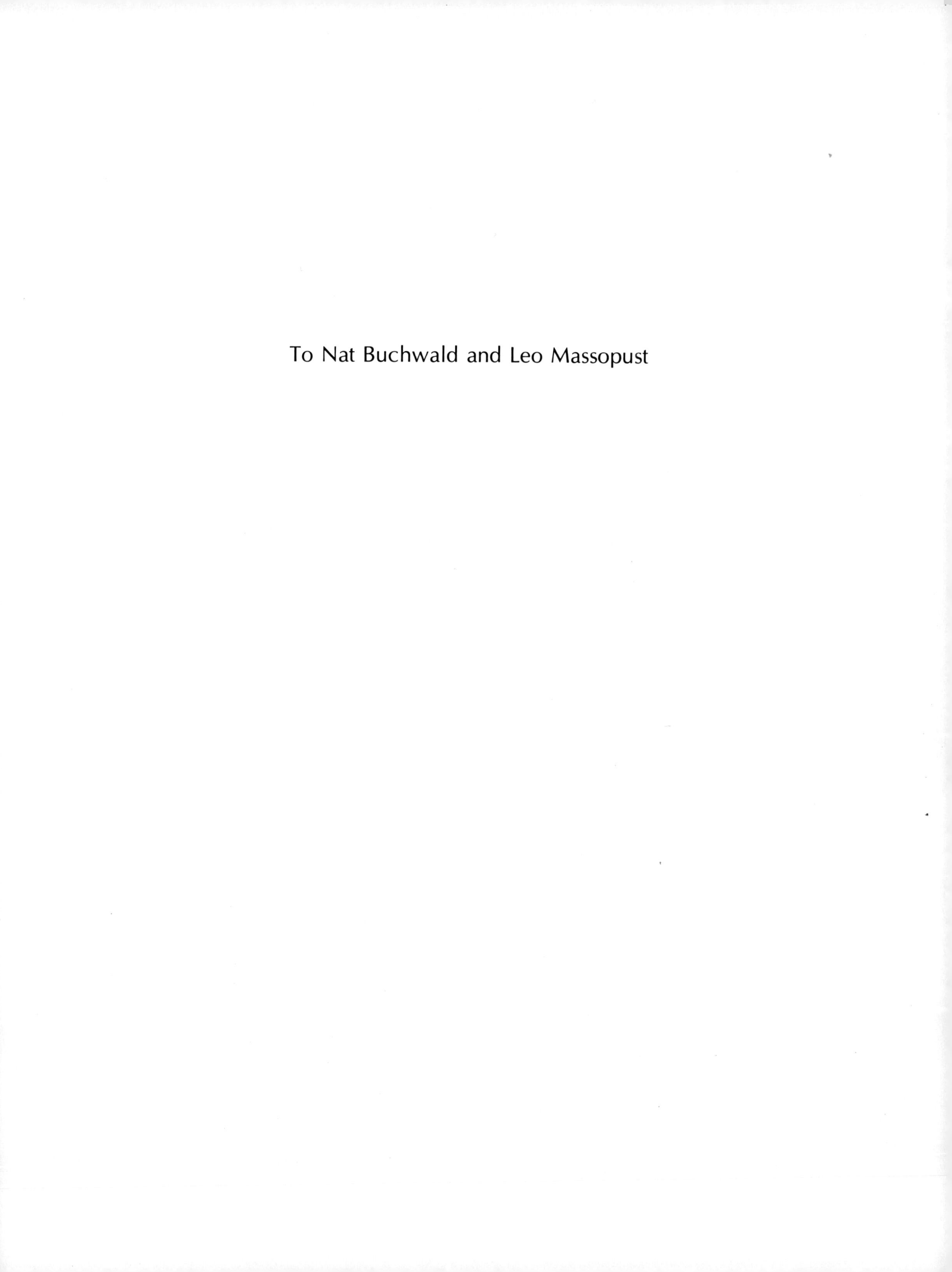

To Nat Buchwald and Leo Massopust

PREFACE

One of the goals of physiological psychology is to discover the neural substrates of behavior. In an effort to achieve this, many researchers have used the method of producing lesions in specific parts of the brain and evaluating the resulting behavioral syndromes. In view of the established value and continued usefulness of this method, there is a need in the neurosciences for a volume providing a comprehensive description of behavioral syndromes arising from local lesions in different parts of the brain. At present, such information is largely confined to clinical neurology texts and is restricted to those syndromes associated with brain lesions in humans. While this is useful to clinicians, it is less than satisfactory for those learning about, reviewing, or conducting neuropsychological research with animals. Differences in the neuropsychological tests used; variations in the size, locus, and origin of the lesions; and the phylogenetic distance between animals and humans make for discrepancies between syndromes described in the clinical and experimental literature.

This book provides a description of the behavioral disturbances in the albino rat that are associated with circumscribed lesions in different parts of the brain. It is a record of personal observations of brain-damaged rats extending over the past 17 years rather than a compilation of the syndromes reported in the literature. This is not to depreciate the various syndromes that have already been described. Many of the published descriptions of behavioral disturbances in the brain-damaged rat (or cat or monkey) have considerable precision and reliability. But it is usually the case that one investigator focuses his attention on one particular part of the brain and on one behavioral process, while a second concentrates on another brain area and an altogether different behavioral process. Since each investigator utilizes a different set of behavioral tests, it is often difficult to compare one syndrome with another. This problem does not arise in connection with the observations reported here because the same behavioral tests were administered to animals with lesions in different parts of the brain. Lesions were placed in 50 different cortical and subcortical structures and 22 different behavioral and physiological "tests" were administered. The latter ranged from retention of previously learned laboratory tasks to observations on activity, aggressiveness, pupil size, and mortality rate.

Choosing the albino rat as a vehicle to develop a compilation of behavioral syndromes needs no apology. In the United States, the rat has been one of the more popular laboratory animals used in neurobehavioral investigations. In fact, much of what is known about the neural substrates of behavior is based on, or at least supplemented by, observations on the rat.

This book should be of use to those who are engaged in neurobehavioral research. It will be of particular interest to the increasing number of investigators who are searching for neurophysiological correlates of behavior or correspondences between the recently described chemical (and anatomical) pathways of the brain and behavior. Students and instructors in physiological psychology or biopsychology courses may also find the book informative, especially when a question arises concerning the behavioral consequences of a lesion to a neural structure that is not given detailed discussion in whatever textbook they are using. And finally, it is certain to be of interest to any reader who tends to take an extreme position in connection with the localization versus nonlocalization (equipotentiality) controversy.

As might be expected, a project of this magnitude could not have been accomplished without the help of research assistants and graduate students. I am especially indebted to those students at Louisiana State University who spent at least one year in my laboratory. Among these students (listed in chronological order) are: Tom Breen, James McNew, Terry Truax, Arlene Schweigerdt, Michael Thorne, Sam Craddock, Lois Stratton, Peter Spiliotis, Ted Petit, Marsha Howze, Joe LeDoux, John Pucheu, Ben McMath, Blue Douglas, Gregory Sisk, and Richard Maples.

The support given me by LSU in the form of grants and sabbatical leaves has been invaluable. Particular gratitude is extended to Dean Irwin A. Berg and Professor Lawrence Seigel for their continued support of my lesion research.

And finally, I wish to pay tribute to my wife, Pitsa, for her patience and love.

Baton Rouge, Louisiana
January 25, 1978

R.T.

CONTENTS

A BEHAVIORAL ATLAS
OF THE RAT BRAIN

1. INTRODUCTION

The analysis of behavioral changes associated with brain damage in animals and humans is one of the oldest and most widely used methods in neuropsychology. In the laboratory situation, this technique, commonly called the ablation or lesion method, is a straightforward approach to acquiring clues about the functional significance of discrete areas of the brain. Assuming that an investigator has focused his attention on the possible functions of a given structure that is within the hypothalamus, for instance, no approach is simpler or more to the point than to destroy that structure in a laboratory animal and observe the subsequent behavior of the animal in a variety of situations. Similarly, if a researcher is interested in finding out what parts of the cerebral cortex are essential for the performance of a particular behavioral act, the most direct approach would be to damage different parts of the neocortex in different animals and then test for the integrity of the behavioral act under investigation.

Like all neuropsychological methods used in the experimental laboratory, the lesion method has its weaknesses (see Section 6), the most conspicuous of which is the uncertainty involved in interpreting the behavioral or physiological changes following local brain damage. In research on memory, for example, it is often difficult to determine whether a lesion-induced amnesia is due to a disturbance in emotionality, motivation, sensory capacities, or storage (Isaacson, 1976). Another weakness of the method is that lesions may produce morphological, physiological, and biochemical alterations in brain areas far removed from the site of the lesion (Lynch, 1976). The possibility exists, therefore, that these "distance effects" initiated by a lesion may contribute significantly more to the appearance of behavioral changes than simple loss of neural tissue.

Despite these weaknesses, the method of ablation has yielded findings which have contributed immensely to our understanding of human brain function, particularly by helping to establish that some parts of the brain are more important for the expression of certain behaviors than are others (see Zülch, Creutzfeldt, & Galbraith, 1975). From a historical point of view, the most notable contribution of these findings bears upon the "localization versus nonlocalization" controversy (Young, 1970). Are discrete physiological, behavioral, and/or mental functions related to the activities of relatively specific parts of the brain or are they products of the activity of the brain as a whole? While some issues concerning this controversy remain unresolved, few would dispute that cerebral localization has been a guiding force in contemporary brain research and that the findings derived from the lesion method provide strong empirical support for that theory.

This is not to say that neuroscientists who are currently using the lesion method (or any other method) have returned to the phrenological viewpoint that for every function there is a corresponding area of the brain whose activity is uniquely specialized for the expression of that function. This extreme position on the localization versus nonlocalization controversy has largely given way to the view that discrete physiological, behavioral, and mental functions depend upon the combined activities of nuclear groups whose elements may be situated at widely dispersed regions throughout the neuraxis (Luria, 1966). Current textbooks of physiological psychology clearly reflect this viewpoint by referring frequently to anatomical systems (as opposed to anatomical "centers") thought to mediate different functions. Some of the more prominent of these systems are the retino-geniculo-striate system governing detail vision, the limbic system mediating emotional experience and behavior, the ascending brainstem reticular system regulating attention and arousal, and the medial forebrain bundle system subserving reward and pleasure.

So long as the anatomical limits of putative functional systems within the brain remain obscure or ill-defined, there will be a need in the neurosciences for additional data derived from the lesion method. Such data can also be useful in locating points of interaction between functional systems and in testing neurological theories concerned with these points of interaction. In addition, lesion experiments are of considerable value to neurophysiologists, neurohistologists, and neurochemists as a source of information about those regions of the brain that are most likely to contain neurons whose physiological, structural, and chemical properties will change in the presence (or absence) of certain kinds of stimulation. And despite the failure so far to locate brain regions that contain the engrams of experience, lesion studies may still hold promise in this quest.

To write a comprehensive review of the behavioral consequences of lesions to different parts of the brain would be a prodigious undertaking. Literally thousands of articles on this subject can be found in the literature. Even if the attempt were made, it is doubtful whether any significant degree of consensus could be arrived at concerning the specific neurological deficits or behavioral syndromes associated with damage to each area of the brain considered. Anyone casually acquainted with the field immediately recognizes the contradictions, confusion, and abundance of theory. This state of confusion has developed largely because so many variables influence the behavioral outcome of local brain damage. Among these variables are the nature, size, and locus of the lesions; the use of one-stage versus two-stage surgical procedures; the length of the recovery period; the species, age, and previous experience of the animal; the conditions of observation; and the criteria used for the determination of a behavioral deficit. If the behavioral test includes the retention of a learned response, then additional variables would come into play, such as the nature of the learned response, the motivation employed, the number of trials given daily, and the criterion of learning.

If descriptions of syndromes associated with lesions to many different areas of the brain are to have any heuristic value, not to mention a significant degree of reliability and validity, they must be based not only upon one particular species of a given age and experience, but upon conditions of observation that are relatively uniform from one brain-damaged animal to the next. To a large degree, the syndromes presented in this volume in the form of maps of specific behavioral and physiological deficits meet these requirements.

Over a number of years, I have had the opportunity to observe more than 2000 rats with lesions in different parts of the brain. In some animals, the lesions were localized to different portions of the neopallium. In others, subcortical formations ranging from the septal area to the pontine reticular formation were discretely damaged. Many of these rats were observed both ''semiformally'' on an observation table and formally within specially constructed apparatuses designed to study learning and retention of learning.

Since most of the observations were made personally, a certain bias pervading the data cannot be denied, especially in relation to the semiformal tests of behavioral disturbances. In most of the rats studied, I was aware of the intended locus of the lesions. This knowledge, combined with certain expectations about the behavioral outcome of specific lesions (gained through repeated experience with rats having similar parts of the brain destroyed), would clearly have an influence upon which disturbances were detected and which ones were undetected. To what extent these expectations influenced the pattern of deficits observed with each brain lesion I cannot judge. However, one detail must be mentioned which may have, at least in part, neutralized this bias. This is the fact that the intended site of the lesion and its verified site (discovered through the use of histological controls) may be astonishingly distant from each other. With present stereotaxic techniques, inaccuracies in the placement of lesions occur frequently enough to prevent investigators (including myself) from relying upon the stereotaxic coordinates for the position and size of a lesion.

Because differences in methodology often lead to differences in the composition of syndromes, it will be necessary to discuss in some detail the procedures that were used in gathering the data that will be presented graphically in a later section of this book.

PLAN OF THE BOOK

In Section 2 details about the animals, behavioral methods (tests), and surgical and histological procedures are given.

Section 3 describes the manner in which the results were mapped on brain sections.

Section 4 presents the illustrations that constitute the main body of data. At the beginning of the section there is a list of brain structures where the lesions were placed. Each line drawing of a brain section showing the site of the lesion and its associated syndrome is accompanied by a photograph of a corresponding unstained brain section appropriately labeled and furnished with frontal, lateral, and vertical stereotaxic coordinates scaled in millimeters. These illustrations are organized in a manner similar to that of a stereotaxic atlas. The first diagram presents the cerebral surface along with the sites of lesions to the cerebral surface, olfactory bulbs, and cerebellum. This is followed by a diagram of a parasagittal section of the brain showing the locus and extent of damage to two separate regions of the cingulate (limbic) cortex. In subsequent illustrations, diagrams of frontal sections through the brainstem are used to depict the sites of lesions to the various structures located within the interior parts of the brain. These frontal sections proceed from anterior to posterior levels.

It is possible to cast the lesion data presented in Section 4 into maps of specific deficits. This can be done by plotting the distribution of lesions that produced the same specific deficit (e.g., aggressiveness). Since 22 different behavioral and physiological deficits were recorded, 22 maps would result. At the beginning of Section 5 there is a list of the specific deficits along with the number of the figure (a parasagittal section) that provides the corresponding map. The maps referring to specific deficits follow. These maps are a unique source of clues concerning the functional and anatomical relationships existing among different parts of the brain.

Section 6 discusses some of the problems related to the interpretation of lesion data and describes the limited inferences that can be made about the functions of specific brain structures. Some comments on the interpretation of the results presented in Sections 4 and 5 are also included.

Finally, a list of suggested readings is provided for those who wish to pursue the functional anatomy of the behavioral and physiological responses investigated in this monograph.

2. GENERAL METHODS

RATS

Only adult male laboratory rats (*Rattus norvegicus* var. *albinus*) of the Wistar strain were used. In most cases, these animals were born and reared in the vivarium at the Louisiana State University psychology laboratory. When selected for study, the animals weighed from 400 to 650 g. They were usually housed two per cage in medium-size wire cages containing a constant supply of food pellets and water. Before its assignment to experimental training on any one of the learning tasks to be described below, each rat was handled periodically and allowed to explore the surface of a black masonite table. Those rats showing signs of eye disease, middle-ear infection, or any other neurological disorders were discarded. Also discarded were rats that persisted in showing aggression toward the experimenter or toward their cage mates.

After being trained on a particular learning problem, most of the rats sustained bilateral cortical or subcortical lesions, and were subsequently tested for retention of learning that problem after an interval of 2–3 weeks. The rats that did not receive brain damage served as controls and were of two types: unoperated (normal) controls and sham-operated controls. The sham-operated rats underwent the same surgical procedures as the brain-damaged rats (anesthetization, shaving of hair over cranium, placement into a headholder, longitudinal incision across the cranium, reflection of underlying tissues, drilling of holes into the skull, suturing of the skin, and application of 3% Aureomycin ointment over the wound), except for insertion of a lesion electrode or suction tube into the brain. (Since the sham-operated and normal control rats were virtually indistinguishable from each other on the behavioral and physiological tests administered in this investigation, the syndromes presented in Section 4 can be attributed to the induction of brain damage and not to the surgical procedures themselves.)

SURGERY

Surgery was performed under deep chloral hydrate anesthesia. From a mixture of chloral hydrate crystals and water at a concentration of 50 mg/cc, the rat was administered intraperitoneally 2.2–3.0 cc of the chloral hydrate solution. This dose usually produced an anesthetized state within 2 min: righting reflexes were abolished and tail pinch or insertion into the headholder failed to evoke any physical reaction. In some cases, however, injection of an additional 1.0 cc was necessary in order to anesthetize the animal fully.

In most instances, bilateral damage to a given cortical or subcortical area was accomplished in one stage. Two-stage operations (unilateral lesion followed by a contralateral lesion with an interoperative period of 7–10 days) were routinely performed to damage the caudoputamen or globus pallidus and were occasionally performed to damage the red nucleus, substantia nigra, or paramedial portions of the midbrain reticular formation. Two-stage operations were performed on the caudoputamen and globus pallidus in order to reduce the severity and duration of aphagic-adipsic disturbances and on the midbrain areas in order to increase the likelihood of survival beyond the first 48 hr.

Destruction of the olfactory bulbs, neocortical areas, cingulate cortex, or cerebellum was achieved by the aspiration method, using techniques similar to those described by Meyer and Meyer (1971). All other lesions were made stereotaxically (using techniques described by Thompson, 1971) with reference to a modified version of the rat atlas of Massopust (1961). (This version of the Massopust atlas, showing the placement of the lesions and the resulting syndromes, constitutes Section 4, and the directions for its use are presented in Section 3.) Depending on the area to be destroyed, a constant anodal current of 1.5–5.0 milliamperes was passed for 5–15 sec through an implanted stainless steel electrode with 1.0–2.0 mm of the tip exposed. Three types of electrocoagulative lesions were made. Type I lesions were made by a single insertion of the electrode into the brain and the application of current. This type of lesion was routinely made to destroy the interpedunculo-central tegmental (and median raphe) area and occasionally made to destroy the septal area, central gray, or mamillary bodies. Type II lesions involved bilateral destruction of an area through insertion of an electrode on one side to produce a lesion, and then repetition of the procedure on the contralateral side. Most of the subcortical lesions were induced in this manner. Type III lesions were the result of multiple insertions of an electrode on each side for the purpose of enlarging the overall size of the lesions. The brain regions regularly damaged in this manner included the caudoputamen, globus pallidus, dorsal hippocampus, anterior thalamus, superior colliculus, inferior colliculus, subcollicular tegmentum, lateral lemniscal area, and entorhino-subicular area.

A brief description of the surgical steps followed to produce lesions will be given. (For further details, the reader may consult the following sources: Hart, 1976; Skinner, 1971; Singh & Avery, 1975; Thompson, 1971; Webster, 1975.)

1. After the rat was anesthetized, the hair over the cranium was closely shaved with electric clippers.
2. The head of the animal was positioned in the headholder and the shaved portion of the cranium was painted with tincture of Merthiolate.
3. A longitudinal incision was made with a scalpel, starting at eye-level and proceeding posteriorly to include skin half way down the neck. The tissues over the skull were reflected laterally with the handle end of the scalpel. In some cases, forceps were used to keep the skin flaps retracted. Gauze pads were used to remove any blood from the exposed surface of the skull.
4. When cortex, olfactory bulb, or cerebellum was the target for ablation, small holes were made in the skull overlying the appropriate brain area with an electric drill. These holes were then widened with rongeurs. The dura was cut with a needle and retracted with forceps. With the use of a portable aspirator and a #18-gauge hypodermic needle (the tip being blunted) fitted into the rubber suction tubing, the target area was removed.
5. When subcortical lesions were desired, small holes were made in the skull where the lesion electrode would be inserted. With the use of a stereotaxic instrument, the lesion electrode was lowered into the brain. From the lesion-maker, the anodal lead was attached to the electrode, and the cathodal lead was clamped to the exposed muscles of the neck. The current was then applied.
6. When all bleeding stopped, the skin was sutured with 9-mm wound clips. Aureomycin ointment was applied liberally to the surface of the wound.

POSTOPERATIVE CARE

Immediately after surgery, the animal was placed into a separate cage containing neither food nor water. Since the anesthetic used (chloral hydrate) is short-lasting, no special effort was made to keep the animal warm during the period of anesthetization. Water and food were made available 24 hr after surgery.

During the first few postoperative days, each rat was allowed to recover in a separate cage, but at least one week before the retention test it was paired with another operated (or control) rat. However, those rats that failed to regain normal eating and drinking habits were kept in isolation and provided with one or more dishes of fresh wet mash daily. If the aphagia and adipsia continued, the retention test was usually initiated at the end of the first postoperative week.

Throughout the postoperative period, observations of the general behavior of each rat were made on the black masonite table.

HISTOLOGY

At the conclusion of all postoperative testing, each brain-damaged rat was killed with an overdose of Nembutal, its vascular system perfused with normal saline followed by 10% formalin, and the brain removed and stored in 10% formalin for 2–7 days. For neocortical injuries, the lesion was reconstructed on Lashley-type brain diagrams before sectioning.

With a freezing microtome, each brain was sectioned frontally at 90 microns in the stereotaxic plane of Massopust (1961). Every third section showing the lesion was photographed at 10–14X by using the unstained section as a negative film in an enlarger (see Thompson, 1971). These photographs of unstained sections yield differentiation of the brain field similar to that obtained with a fiber stain and readily permit identification of the three major zones of the lesion—the vacuolated area, the narrow rim of severely coagulated tissue, and the surrounding gliosis (see Fig. 2-1).

While this method of verifying the locus and extent of the lesions does not provide the finer detail obtained with more customary histological techniques, it serves most satisfactorily as a "screening" device to separate rats into various groups according to the principal site of the lesions.

BEHAVIORAL TESTS AND DEFICITS

1. Visual discrimination habits. Over 600 rats were trained on a brightness discrimination task (white card positive, black card negative), a pattern discrimination task (horizontal black- and white-striped card positive, vertical black- and white-striped card negative), or both in a two-choice discrimination apparatus (Thompson & Bryant, 1955). Figure 2-2 shows the discrimination apparatus. Under the motive of escape from (or avoidance of) footshock, each rat was trained to approach and displace the positive stimulus card and to avoid the adjacent negative stimulus card. The position of the positive card was switched from right to left either in a strict double-alternation sequence or in a sequence mixed with single- and double-alternation runs. A response to the unlocked positive card (correct response) admitted the rat to the goal box, whereas a response to the locked negative card (error) was followed by the automatic administration of mild footshock. Eight trials were given daily with an intertrial interval of 60 sec. Fifteen correct responses on two consecutive days constituted the criterion of learning. After learning the tasks, most of the rats were subjected to cortical or subcortical lesions.

The retention test, which consisted of relearning the problem (or problems), utilized the same procedures as the original test. The retention measure was expressed in terms of conventional percentage error savings scores which relate the individual relearning score with the corresponding original learning score.

In terms of savings scores, three general outcomes are possible. First, the brain-damaged rat may relearn the problem about as fast as the normal (or sham-operated) controls and, as a consequence, achieve a high positive savings score—80% of the control rats earned savings scores in excess of 90%. Second, the brain-damaged animal may show some transient difficulty in regaining the habit, but then relearn at a faster rate than in original learning. In this case, the savings score will be lower

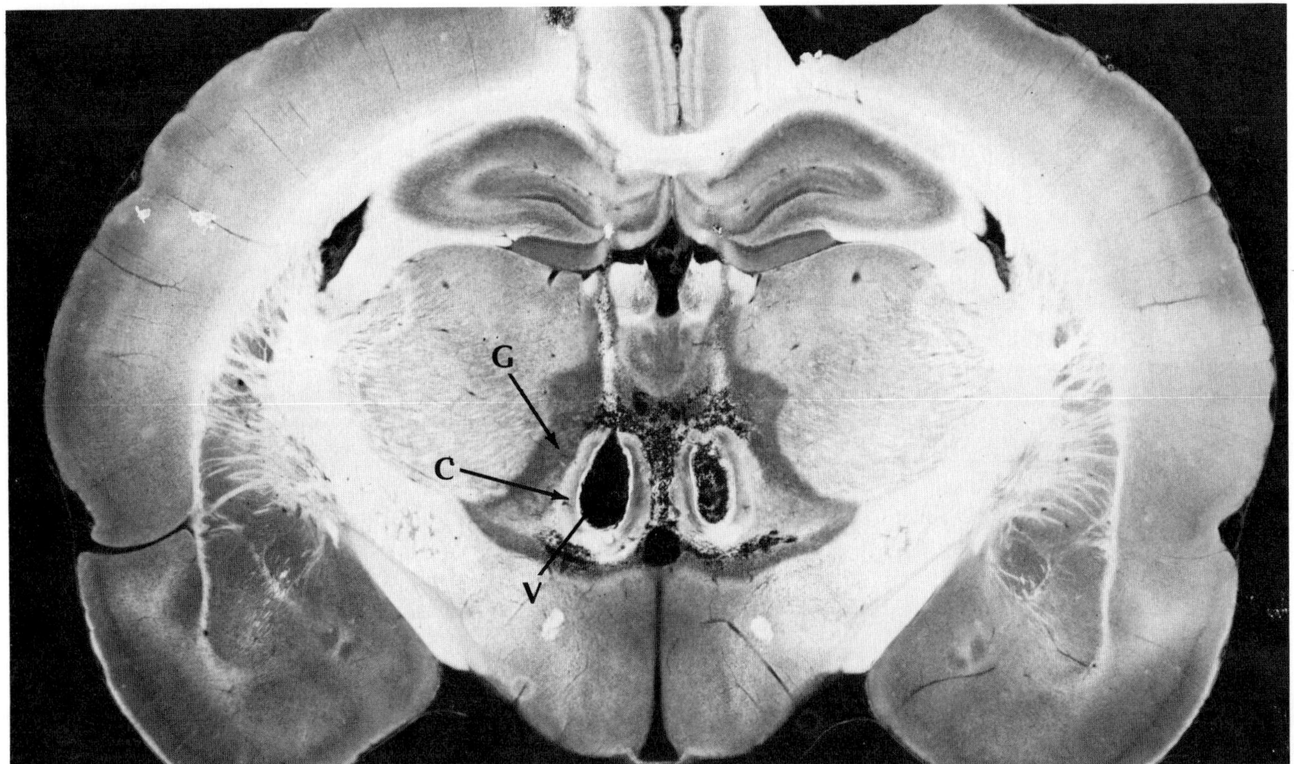

Fig. 2-1. Photograph of an unstained brain section showing a lesion (Type II) to the ventromedial thalamus. Note the three zones of the lesion—vacuolated area (**V**), narrow rim of severely coagulated tissue (**C**), and gliosis (**G**). The central necrotic zone of the lesion consists of the areas occupied by **V** and **C** only.

than that associated with the first outcome, but still of positive sign. Finally, the brain-damaged rat may show an enduring disturbance in reaching the criterion to the degree that the problem is relearned at a similar or slower rate. In this case, the savings score will be zero or negative. Since the poorest control animal earned a positive savings score (30%), there is little doubt that a zero or negative savings score reflects a serious disturbance in the expression of the visual discrimination habit. *Thus, any brain-damaged rat earning a zero or negative savings score on either the brightness or pattern task was considered to show a visual discrimination deficit.*

2. Vestibulo-kinesthetic discrimination habit. Over 400 blinded rats were trained to choose an upward sloping arm and to avoid a downward sloping arm in a single-unit T-maze adapted for the use of escape from footshock as a motive

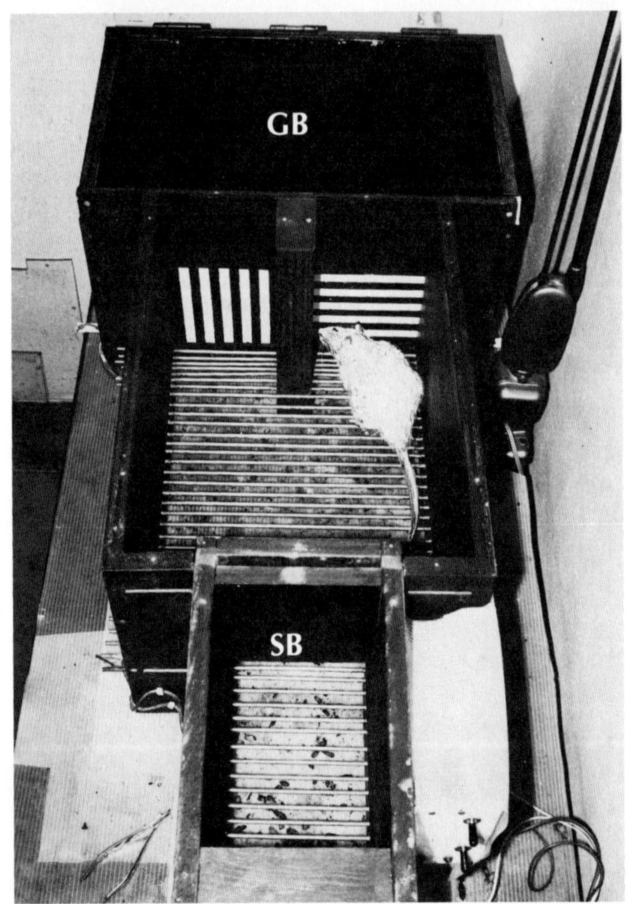

Fig. 2-2. Photograph of the visual discrimination apparatus showing the start box (**SB**), choice chamber, discriminanda, and goal box (**GB**).

5

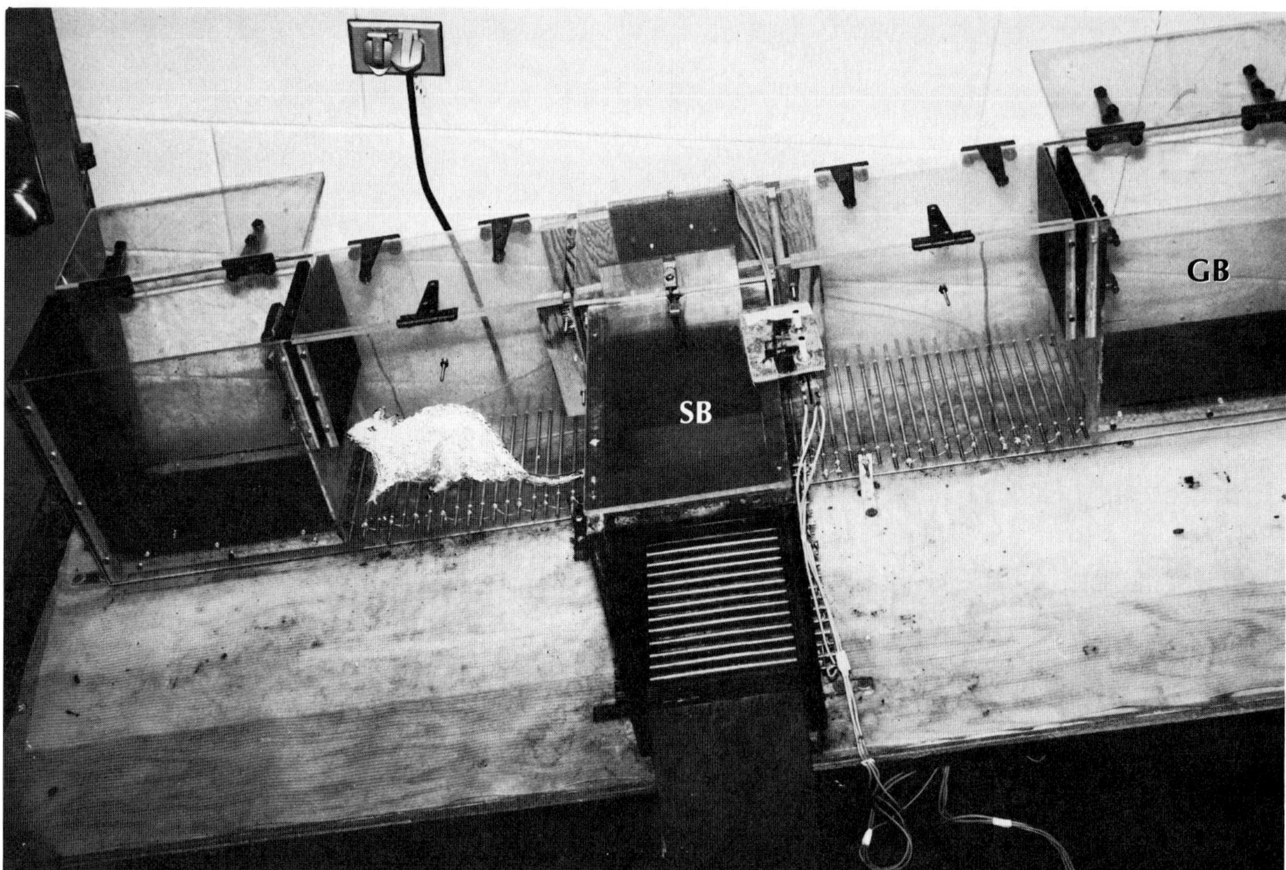

Fig. 2-3. Photograph of the incline plane discrimination apparatus showing the start box (**SB**), arms of the T, and the goal box (**GB**).

(Thompson et al., 1961). This apparatus is shown in Figure 2-3. The correct arm led to an endbox which could be entered by knocking down an unlocked card. The incorrect arm led to a locked card that prevented the rat from entering the endbox on that side. The position of the correct arm was switched from right to left in an order mixed with single- and double-alternation runs. Punishment for errors was given by electric charge through the grid section located in front of the locked card. Six to eight trials were given daily with an intertrial interval of 60 sec. No more than one error in two consecutive days constituted the criterion of learning. After the criterion had been met, most of the rats received cortical or subcortical lesions.

As in the visual discrimination situation, the retention test consisted of relearning the habit and the measure of retention was expressed in terms of percentage error savings scores. Again, a zero or negative savings score would reflect a serious deficit in the expression of the vestibulo-kinesthetic habit; the poorest control animal earned a positive score (50%). *Thus, any brain-damaged rat earning a zero or negative savings score was considered to show a vestibulo-kinesthetic discrimination deficit.*

3. Card displacement habit. All rats required to learn either the visual or vestibulo-kinesthetic discrimination tasks were initially trained in the corresponding apparatus to push aside a gray card in order to gain access to the goal box. This habit is readily learned, requiring no more than a dozen trials. At the outset, each card was positioned at a 45° angle from the window, allowing a space for the rat to enter the goal box from the choice chamber (or arm of the T). On subsequent trials, the card was positioned at a smaller angle from the window. Card displacement training was terminated after the rat displaced the card on three successive trials when the card was in a position flush against the window. Well over 90% of the rats pushed open the card with their nose; the rest used their forepaws.

Once acquired, this card displacement habit is retained by control rats for several months with virtually no forgetting. Blinding the rat does not abolish the habit. Some brain-damaged rats, however, do display a disturbance of this habit. (In such a case, the experimenter would displace the card to allow the rat to enter the goal box.) Thus, *any brain-damaged rat failing to push aside the card on at least half of the trials during the first postoperative test day was considered to show a card displacement deficit.*

4. Maze habit. Over 300 rats were trained on a three-cul maze which was adapted for the use of escape from footshock as a motive (Thompson, 1974). This maze is shown in Figure

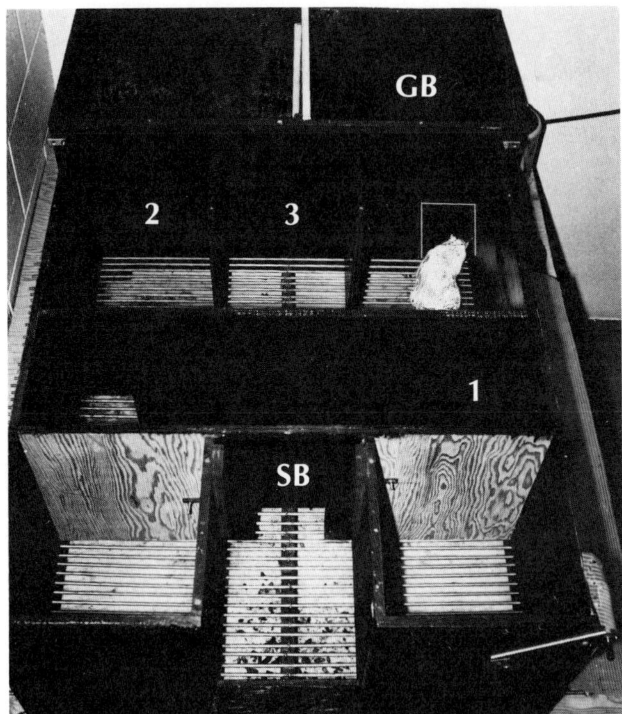

Fig. 2-4. Photograph of the maze showing the start box (**SB**), the three blind alleys (**1**, **2**, and **3**), and the goal box (**GB**).

2-4. An error was defined as entering the blind alley by at least the length of the rat's head and thorax. Only initial errors were recorded—the animal could make no more than three errors per trial. Four trials were given daily with an intertrial interval of 75 sec. Two consecutive errorless days constituted the criterion of learning. After learning had been accomplished, most of the animals were subjected to either cortical or subcortical damage.

The retention test consisted of relearning the maze, and the retention measure involved the use of percentage error savings. The poorest control animal earned a savings score of 50%. *Thus, any brain-damaged rat earning a zero or negative savings score was considered to show a maze deficit.*

5. Active avoidance habit. More than 300 rats were trained to jump out of a box within 10 sec in order to avoid footshock. The area of safety was a ledge which rimmed the perimeter of the box. This apparatus, shown in Figure 2-5, is similar to that described ay Maatsch (1959). If the rat failed to make the jumping response within 10 sec (error), footshocks were administered at a rate of about one every two seconds until the appropriate jumping response was made. Shock intensity averaged 2.5 milliamperes. One trial was given daily for 10 consecutive days. Following training, the majority of rats sustained either cortical or subcortical lesions.

The postoperative test consisted of 10 trials administered at a rate of one trial per day. Since no predetermined criterion of learning was used in this experiment, it was necessary to establish an arbitrary criterion in order to compute a savings score. The first appearance of an avoidance response was chosen as the criterion of learning (and relearning). In this case, the number of errors (trials) made before the first appearance of an avoidance response in the original learning period was compared with the number of errors before the first appearance of an avoidance response postoperatively. All control animals earned positive savings scores. *Thus, any brain-damaged rat earning zero or negative savings scores was considered to show an active avoidance response deficit.*

6. Escape response habit. For the active-avoidance conditioning situation described above, the rat's escape response was to jump out of the box after a footshock. (The rat's avoidance response was to jump out of the box prior to the onset of footshock.) This particular response is subject to learning to the extent that about 20 footshocks were necessary to elicit a successful jumping reaction on the first day, about two footshocks were needed on the second day, and an average of less than one footshock was required on the third day—this last result was due to the fact that some rats began making an avoidance response.

The criterion for learning the escape response was arbitrarily defined as the first appearance of a successful jumping response following the application of a single footshock. A savings score could be computed from these data simply by comparing the number of days required to learn the escape response preoperatively with the number of days required to learn the escape response postoperatively. All control animals earned savings scores ranging from 0 to 100%. *Thus, any*

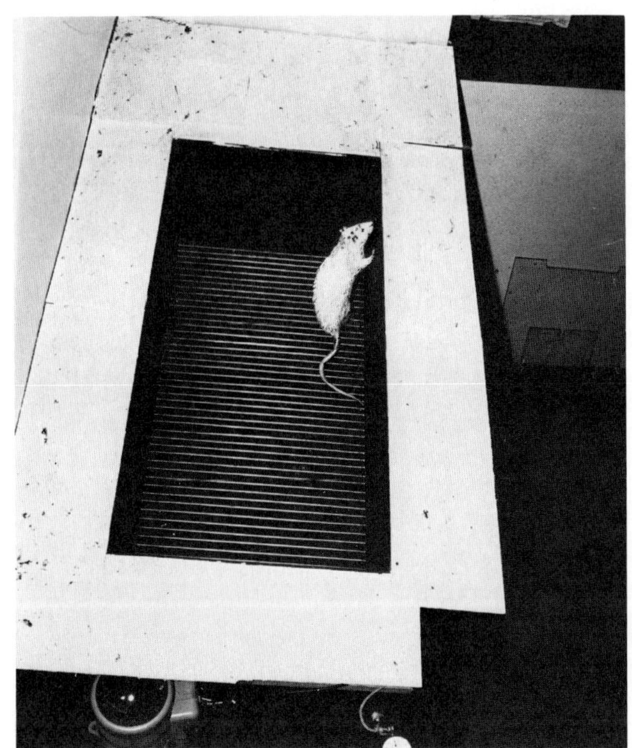

Fig. 2-5. Photograph of the escape avoidance apparatus showing the grid floor and the overlying area of safety (white ledge surrounding the box).

brain-damaged rat earning a negative savings score was considered to show an escape response deficit.

1. "Hypermetamorphosis."   This term is reluctantly used to designate an abnormal exploratory tendency seen in some brain-damaged rats. The decision to resort to the term is based on two compelling parallels. First, the exploratory tendency in some of the brain-damaged rats (to be described below) remarkably resembles that seen in certain brain-damaged monkeys that have been described as showing a "hypermetamorphic impulse to action" (Klüver & Bucy, 1939). Second, the location of brain lesions associated with this exploratory tendency in the rat are not far removed from those in the aforementioned monkeys.

This peculiar exploratory tendency was most frequently observed in the visual discrimination apparatus. When introduced into the start box, the rat would promptly explore the grid floor and wooden walls by sniffing one area after another. Footshocks were applied to force the animal into the choice chamber, but once the footshocks were suspended, the rat would resume sniffing various regions of the floor and walls. This "compulsive" sniffing behavior often persisted for several days and did not readily subside despite the fact that footshocks invariably followed the appearance of this behavior. This kind of reaction was not observed in the control rat during the retention test. *Thus, any brain-damaged rat that persisted in sniffing one section of the apparatus after another on most trials of the first postoperative test day was considered to exhibit the disorder of hypermetamorphosis.*

2. Obstinate progression.   In connection with the discrimination problems and the maze habit, an error consisted of entry into an incorrect section of the apparatus; rats committing such errors were then punished by brief footshocks. In the retention test, the control rat would usually retreat from the incorrect section after receiving one or, at most, two footshocks. Some brain-damaged rats, however, would persist in pushing against the incorrect card (or wall in the case of the maze) despite multiple footshocks and, in addition, would continue to show this obstinacy whenever an error was committed. *Thus, any brain-damaged rat that persisted in pushing against the incorrect card (or wall) despite multiple footshocks on virtually every trial in which an error was committed during the first day of the retention test was considered to exhibit the disorder of obstinate progression.*

As mentioned earlier, observations of the behavior of each brain-damaged rat were made on a black masonite table. In most cases, observations were made every 48 hr, starting on the second day after surgery. Unless specified otherwise, a particular behavioral deficit was ascribed to the animal only if that deficit was consistently observed during the course of the first postoperative week (three separate observations).

1. *Hypokinesia.* When placed on the table, the rat would fail to show any locomotor movements for 60 sec.
2. *Hyperkinesia.* When placed on the table, the rat would proceed to run rapidly for 60 sec. In this case, the tail of the rat was held gently but firmly in order to prevent the animal from falling off the table.
3. *Hypersensitivity.* When the rat's face (left side, then right side) was tapped by the observer's hand, a sharp startle response was elicited.
4. *Aphagia-adipsia.* Despite the presence of soft (and hard) food within the home cage, the rat would show no evidence of eating or drinking and would continue to lose weight during the first postoperative week.
5. *Hyperphagia.* During the second and/or third postoperative week, the rat would assume a strikingly obese appearance. (Weight records were not kept after the animal was judged to be recovering normally from surgery.)
6. *Aggressiveness.* When the observer attempted to remove the rat from its home cage, the rat would attempt to bite. (Only one observation was necessary.)
7. *Jerky head movements* (Parkinsonism). The rat would exhibit either a "tremor at rest" of the head in the horizontal plane or jerky movements of the head in both the horizontal and vertical planes.
8. *Hyperextension of the head.* During quadrupedal locomotion, the animal's head would be extended upward at least 45° from the horizontal plane. (Only one observation was necessary.)
9. *Abnormality of gait.* Forward quadrupedal locomotion would appear uncoordinated. (Only two observations were necessary.)
10. *Somnolence.* The rat would be inactive, assuming a hunched, sleep-like posture, with half-closed eyes.
11. *"Coma."* It was impossible to arouse the rat from sleep by opening the home cage and handling the animal. After being returned to its home cage, the animal was later found to be awake and usually active. (Only one observation was necessary.)
12. *Defective pupilloconstrictor reflex.* In the presence of a bright light the pupils would remain fully dilated.
13. *Defective labyrinthine reflex.* At the conclusion of the retention test, the rat was immersed into a tank of water, and would proceed to tuck its head downward while swimming on or beneath the surface.
14. *High mortality rate.* Death occurred within 48 hr after surgery. (Although not regarded as a deficit, this observation was included for the purpose of examining regional differences in mortality rates following brain damage.)

3. CONSTRUCTION OF THE ATLAS

MODIFIED VERSION OF THE MASSOPUST ATLAS

Since the behavioral atlas is based on a modification and extension of the stereotaxic atlas of the rat brain developed by Massopust (1961), a description of the procedures for its use will be given below. This description does not precisely follow that provided by Massopust because the rats involved in the current investigation weighed over 400 g (Massopust's atlas was based on observations of rats weighing 200–300 g) and because the anterior-posterior (frontal) coordinates used to guide the lesion electrodes were based on the position of lambda (the intersection of the transverse and longitudinal skull sutures—see Fig. 3-1) rather than upon the auditory meatuses, as suggested by Massopust.

The modified version of the Massopust atlas is presented in Section 4 in the form of enlarged photographs of frontal sections of the brain cut in the vertical plane (see Figs. 4-3 to 4-16). The lateral and vertical coordinates are scaled in millimeters. At the top of each photograph, F refers to the level of the frontal section in terms of the distance in millimeters from lambda. Coordinate measurements caudal to lambda are indicated with a minus (–) sign, while those rostral to lambda are given in positive numbers. The specific naming of the nuclei and tracts denoted in the photographs did not follow any particular convention. In most cases, however, the nomenclature was guided by the rat atlases of Massopust (1961) and König and Klippel (1963).

The cardinal difference between stereotaxic atlases of the rat brain lies in the orientation of the head (and brain) with respect to the horizontal axis. The orientation of the head, in turn, is governed by the position of the incisor bar in relation to the ear bars of the headholder. In some atlases (Pellegrino & Cushman, 1967; Skinner, 1971), the rat's head is inclined upward by adjusting the incisor bar above the level of the ear bars. In other atlases (König & Klippel, 1963; Massopust, 1961), the head assumes a more horizontal position because the incisor bar is adjusted below the level of the ear bars. In the modified version of the Massopust atlas shown in Section 4, the incisor bar is adjusted 7.0 mm below the level of the ear bars. This adjustment places the head (and brain) of a 400–600-g rat, for all practical purposes, in a horizontal position.

Thus, use of the stereotaxic atlas presented in Section 4 requires an adjustment of the headholder so that the incisor bar is positioned 7.0 mm below the ear bars. The frontal, lateral, and vertical coordinates may then be used to guide the electrode to any desired brain site. (I have used this atlas with a moderate degree of success for the past decade.)

BEHAVIORAL ANALYSIS

It is not uncommon for two or more rats having strikingly similar lesions to show sharp differences in the degree to which a particular behavioral deficit is expressed. In fact, one rat may display a deficit, while another may display no deficit despite the similarities in the locus and extent of the lesions. For example, one rat with an occipito-temporal ablation may require twice the number of trials to relearn a brightness discrimination task as compared to original learning, while a second occipito-temporalectomized rat may relearn the habit at a faster rate than in original learning. Or one rat with a medial supra-

Fig. 3-1. Photograph of the exposed skull and neck muscles of the rat showing the position of lambda (**L**).

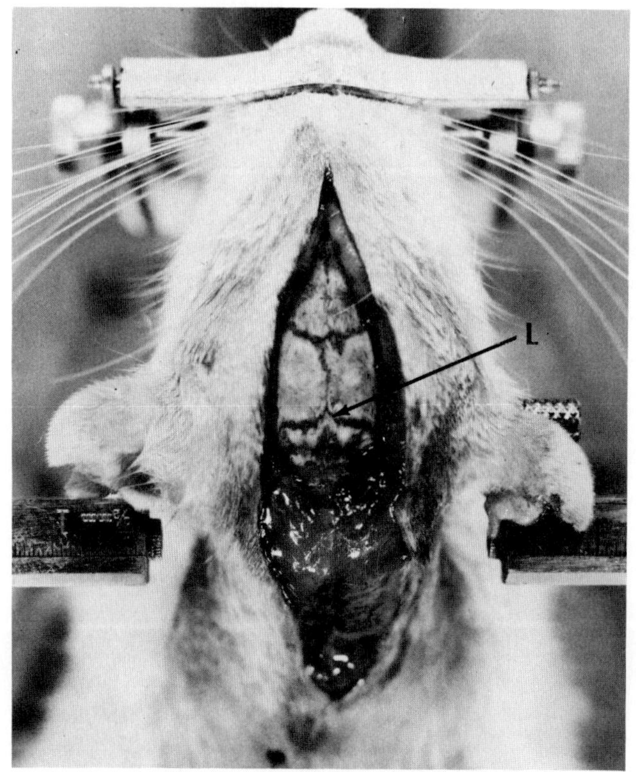

optic hypothalamic lesion may exhibit ferocity evoked by handling, whereas a second rat with a comparable lesion may accept handling with little or no resistance. These differences in the behavioral outcome of brain damage to specific regions may be attributable to subtle differences in the locus, size, and symmetry of the lesion, but other factors may be involved as well.

In the current study, the criterion for including a specific behavioral deficit within a syndrome characteristic of a particular lesion was based on the probability of observing that behavioral deficit in the sample of brain-damaged animals under investigation. This criterion necessarily requires the establishment of an arbitrary cutoff point on the probability scale. It was decided that a specific behavioral deficit which appeared in at least 25% of the cases examined would be included within the syndrome characteristic of that lesion. In order to provide an indication in the atlas as to how frequently the behavioral deficit was observed in the sample of brain-damaged animals examined, the following procedure was used: A deficit that was seen in 25–49% of the cases was listed under the syndrome in light-faced type, a deficit seen in 50–74% of the cases was denoted in italic type, and a deficit seen in 75–100% of the cases was denoted in boldface.

ANATOMICAL ANALYSIS

Well over 1500 brain-damaged rats were observed. Many, however, had to be discarded from consideration in the construction of the atlas because their lesions were unusually small or large, intolerably asymmetrical, or placed within regions which were not intended for study.

For each area of the brain examined, a minimum of 16 animals was used. (More specifically, for each area of the brain examined, a minimum of four animals was used on each of the four major learning tasks—visual discrimination, vestibulo-kinesthetic discrimination, maze, and avoidance habits.) Their lesions to a given brain site, though not identical in locus or magnitude, were similar to the degree that the area of common damage occupied at least 33% of the area of any given individual lesion.

Lesions were placed in three separate regions of the neocortex—the occipito-temporal region, the parietal region, and the frontal region. In Figure 4-1, a "typical" lesion to each of these regions is reconstructed in a schematic drawing of the dorsal surface of the cerebral cortex, and the associated syndrome is noted. (Although all lesions considered in the construction of this atlas were bilateral and reasonably symmetrical, the area of damage is depicted only on the right side of each schematic drawing.)

Two other groups of animals sustained virtually complete ablations of the olfactory bulb and cerebellum, respectively. The syndromes associated with each of these ablations are also noted in the schematic drawing of Figure 4-1.

Two divisions of the cingulate (limbic) cortex were examined: the anterior cingulate area and the posterior cingulate area. A typical ablation of each of these areas and its associated syndrome are presented in a schematic drawing of a parasagittal section of the rat brain (Fig. 4-2). (It should be

noted at this point that the anterior cingulate cortex of the rat may be homologous with the primate prefrontal cortex—see Leonard, 1969.)

The lesions in all remaining areas of the brain are depicted in schematic drawings of frontal sections through the brainstem. Fourteen levels of the brainstem were investigated, corresponding to the 14 frontal sections making up the modified version of the Massopust atlas (see Figs. 4-3 to 4-16). For every area of the brainstem examined, a typical lesion is shown in prominent (heavy) lines and the associated syndrome is noted. The boundaries of each lesion represent only the central necrotic zone; the area of gliosis is not included (see Fig. 2-1). To avoid confusion, a lesion to a given area is depicted on only one frontal section. The section chosen was the one that most closely corresponded to the center of the lesion in all animals of that particular group. It must be emphasized, however, that the lesions almost invariably extended at least 0.5 mm from the center (in both directions) in the rostrocaudal plane, thus damaging, to some degree, structures shown in immediately adjacent frontal sections.

The aspirative ablations as well as the electrolytic lesions presented in this book tend to be larger than those usually reported in the literature. As a result, the lesions are not generally confined to discrete cortical areas, such as Area 17 of Krieg (1946), nor are they limited to discrete subcortical nuclei, such as the nucleus ventralis medialis thalami. Therefore, it was necessary to designate the damaged areas in broad anatomical terms (e.g., occipito-temporal area, ventromedial thalamus). Applying broad anatomical terms to the site of damage is also compatible with the presence of a small but significant degree of intragroup variability both in the size and locus of the lesions.

As mentioned earlier, the photographs of the brain sections (and the respective drawings showing the lesion placements) do not match those presented in more "standard" rat atlases (e.g., König & Klippel, 1963; Pellegrino & Cushman, 1967). Any attempt to reconstruct the lesion placements on a standard atlas would necessarily lead to a small but significant loss in precision in specifying the locus and extent of the damaged area. The reason for this is that electrolytic lesions are usually spherical in shape, and, consequently, would take on a different appearance if illustrated on a frontal section that is in a different plane from the one represented in the modified version of the Massopust atlas. For those who wish to correlate the lesion placements with a standard atlas, however, the one provided by König and Klippel would be the most appropriate since its plane more closely approximates the Massopust plane than that of any other atlas.

MAPPING SPECIFIC DEFICITS

The illustrations included within Section 4 are the main body of data in this behavioral atlas. They clearly show that lesions to different parts of the brain (50 in all) disorganize different constellations of behavior; therefore, they provide unequivocal support for the doctrine of cerebral localization. At the same time, however, they demonstrate that certain behavioral deficits may arise from lesions to more than one part of the brain and that no single lesion has a unique disorganizing effect on a specific behavior. These findings provide striking support for the notion that any given behavioral process depends on the activity of an aggregate (or system) of cell groups whose components may often be widely spaced throughout the neuraxis.

Since it is this latter view that largely dominates the thinking of contemporary neuroscientists, it seemed important to cast the data of the behavioral atlas into maps of specific deficits. This has been done by plotting the distribution of lesions in those groups that exhibited the same specific behavioral or physiological deficit. Since 22 different deficits were investigated, 22 different maps were constructed. These maps are shown in Section 5. Each provides a clue concerning the character of the organization of the neural system governing the expression of the behavioral or physiological process under investigation.

To facilitate an appreciation of the organization of each map of a specific deficit and to permit ready comparisons, all data are plotted on a diagram of the same parasagittal section of the rat brain showing the relative positions of the 50 sites (large open circles) where lesions were separately placed. On each map, those sites that were associated with the same deficit (e.g., maze deficit) are marked. Differential markings used to distinguish deficits that were observed in 75–100% of the cases (dark gray) from those observed in 50–75% (medium gray), or 25–49% (light gray) emphasize the location of possible critical focal areas for the behavioral or physiological process under consideration.

4. LESION PLACEMENTS AND SYNDROMES

LIST OF LESIONS AND CORRESPONDING ILLUSTRATIONS

AREA DAMAGED	ILLUSTRATION NUMBER
Neocortex	
Frontal region	4-1
Parietal region	4-1
Occipito-temporal region	4-1
Other Telencephalic Structures	
Olfactory bulbs	4-1
Cingulate cortex (anterior region)	4-2
Cingulate cortex (posterior region)	4-2
Entorhino-subicular area	4-14
Nucleus accumbens septi	4-3
Septal area	4-4
Hippocampus (dorsal)	4-8
Amygdala	4-7
Caudoputamen (rostral)	4-3
Caudoputamen (middle)	4-4
Globus pallidus area	4-5
Entopeduncular area	4-7
Thalamus	
Anterior region	4-6
Dorsomedial region	4-8
Ventromedial region	4-8
Lateral region	4-8
Ventral region	4-8
Parafascicular area	4-9
Nucleus posterior area	4-9
Lateral geniculate nucleus	4-9
Hypothalamus	
Medial forebrain bundle (rostral)	4-5
Medial forebrain bundle (caudal)	4-9
Supraoptic area (medial)	4-6
Ventromedial area	4-8
Mamillary bodies	4-10
Subthalamus	4-9
Pretectal Area	4-9
Brainstem Reticular Formation	
Mesodiencephalic area (medial)	4-10
Prerubral area	4-11
Suprarubral area	4-12
Supranigral area	4-12
Postrubral area	4-13
Ventrolateral midbrain area	4-13
Pontomesencephalic area (ventromedial)	4-15
Pontine area (medial)	4-16
Other Brainstem Structures	
Superior colliculus	4-11
Inferior colliculus	4-15
Subcollicular tegmentum	4-12
Ventral tegmental area	4-11
Substantia nigra	4-12
Pedunculo-nigral area (lateral)	4-11
Red nucleus area	4-12
Central gray area	4-13
Interpedunculo-central tegmental area	4-12
Raphe area (median)	4-15
Lemniscal midbrain area (lateral)	4-15
Cerebellum	4-1

Fig. 4-1

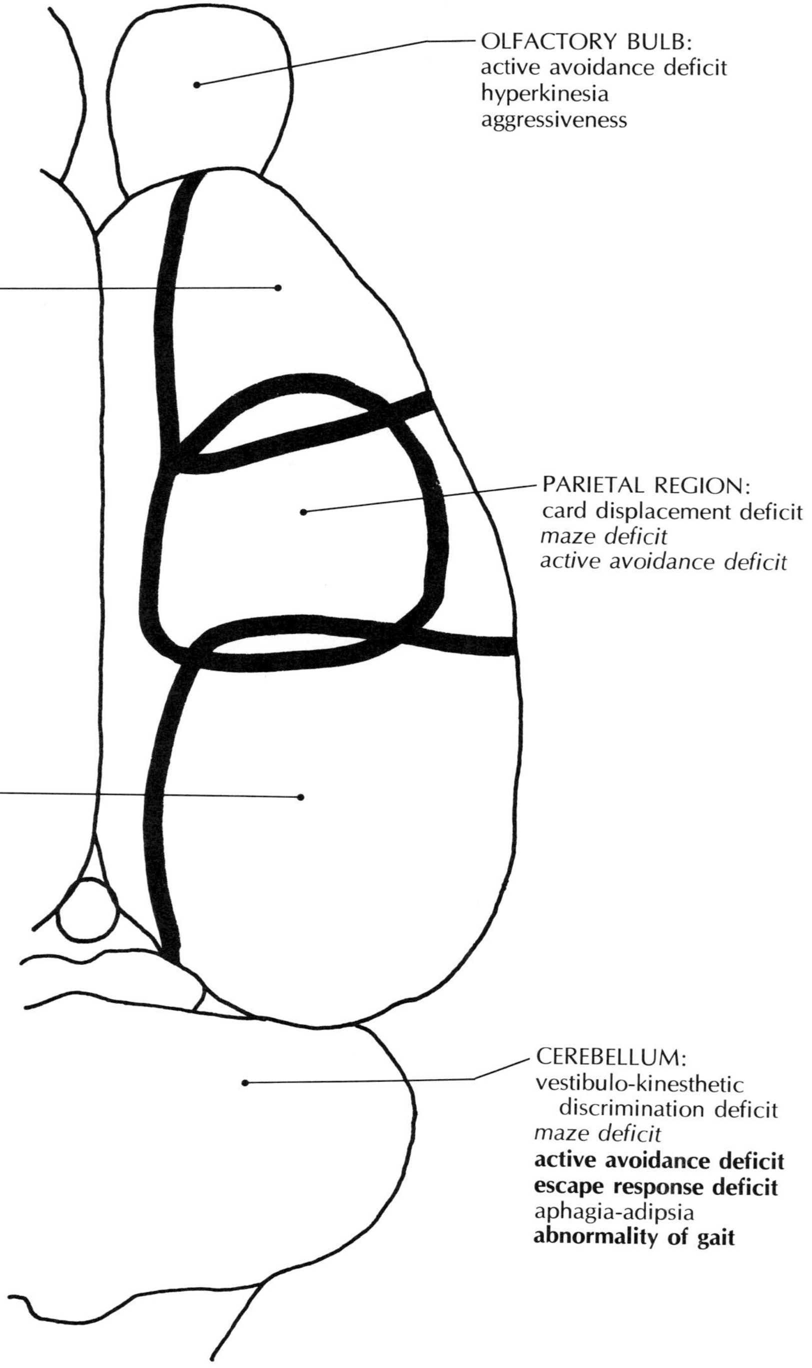

CER—cerebellum
FR—frontal cortex
IC—inferior colliculus
OCC—occipital cortex
OLF—olfactory bulb
PAR—parietal cortex
pi—pineal body
TE—temporal cortex

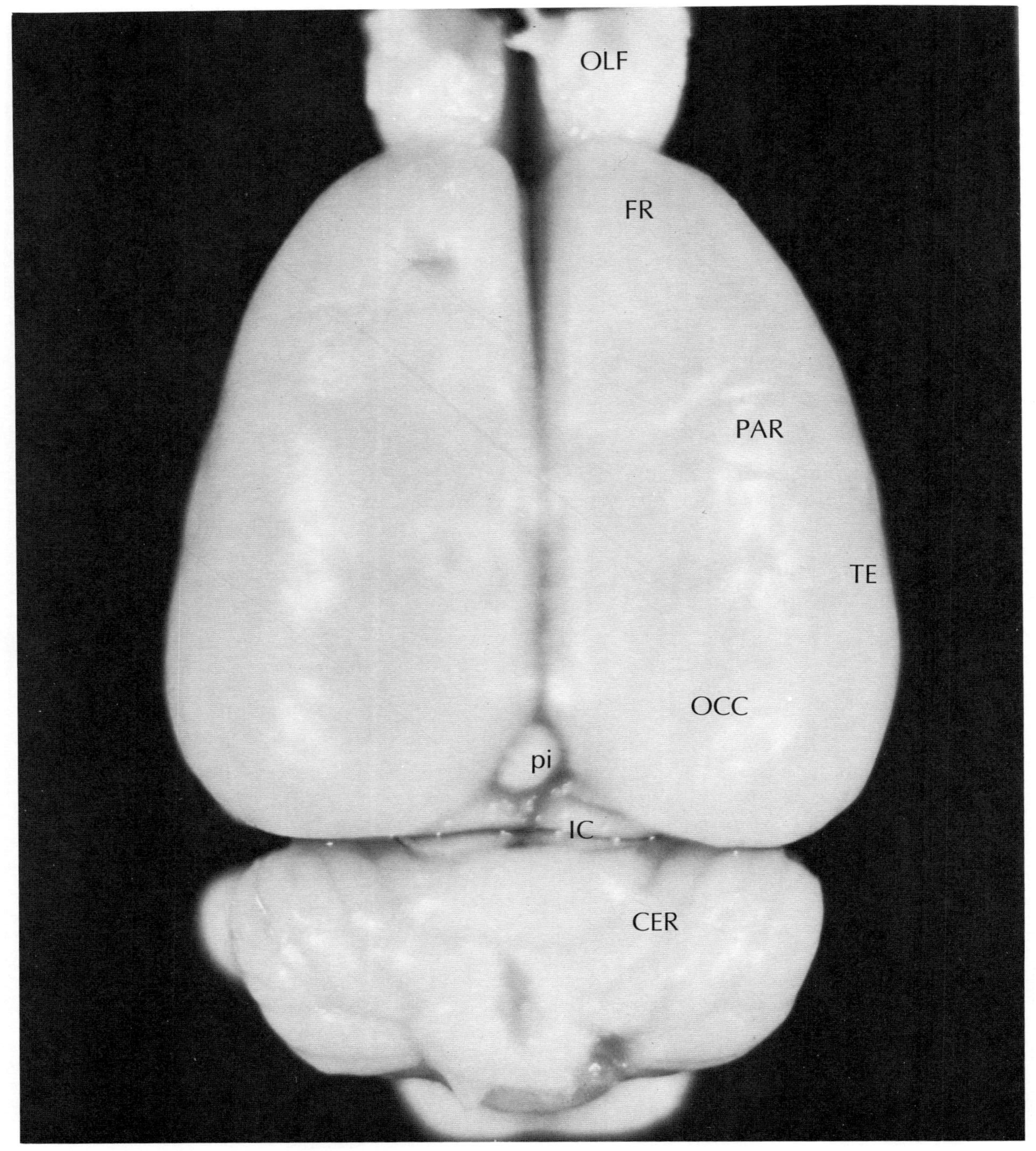

OLF
FR
PAR
TE
OCC
pi
IC
CER

Fig. 4-2

ANTERIOR CINGULATE REGION:
vestibulo-kinesthetic
    discrimination deficit
card displacement deficit
maze deficit
active avoidance deficit
hyperkinesia
hypersensitivity
aggressiveness

POSTERIOR CINGULATE REGION:
vestibulo-kinesthetic
    discrimination deficit
maze deficit

AM—nucleus anterior medialis thalami
CA—anterior commissure
CC—corpus callosum
CER—cerebellum
CG—central gray
DM—nucleus medialis dorsalis thalami
dm—dorsomedial hypothalamic nucleus
F—fornix column
fm—habenulopeduncular tract
HA—anterior hypothalamic nucleus
hab—habenular complex
HIP—hippocampus
IC—inferior colliculus
IR—area infraradiata
mm—medial mamillary nucleus
NAS—nucleus accumbens septi
OLF—olfactory bulb
OPN—optic nerve
P—pons
POM—medial preoptic hypothalamic nucleus
PREC—area precentralis agranularis
r—red nucleus
rpo—nucleus reticularis pontis oralis
RS—area retrosplenialis
SC—superior colliculus
SL—lateral septal nucleus
tpo—nucleus tegmenti pontis
vm—ventromedial hypothalamic nucleus
VM—nucleus ventralis medialis thalami
vta—ventral tegmental area

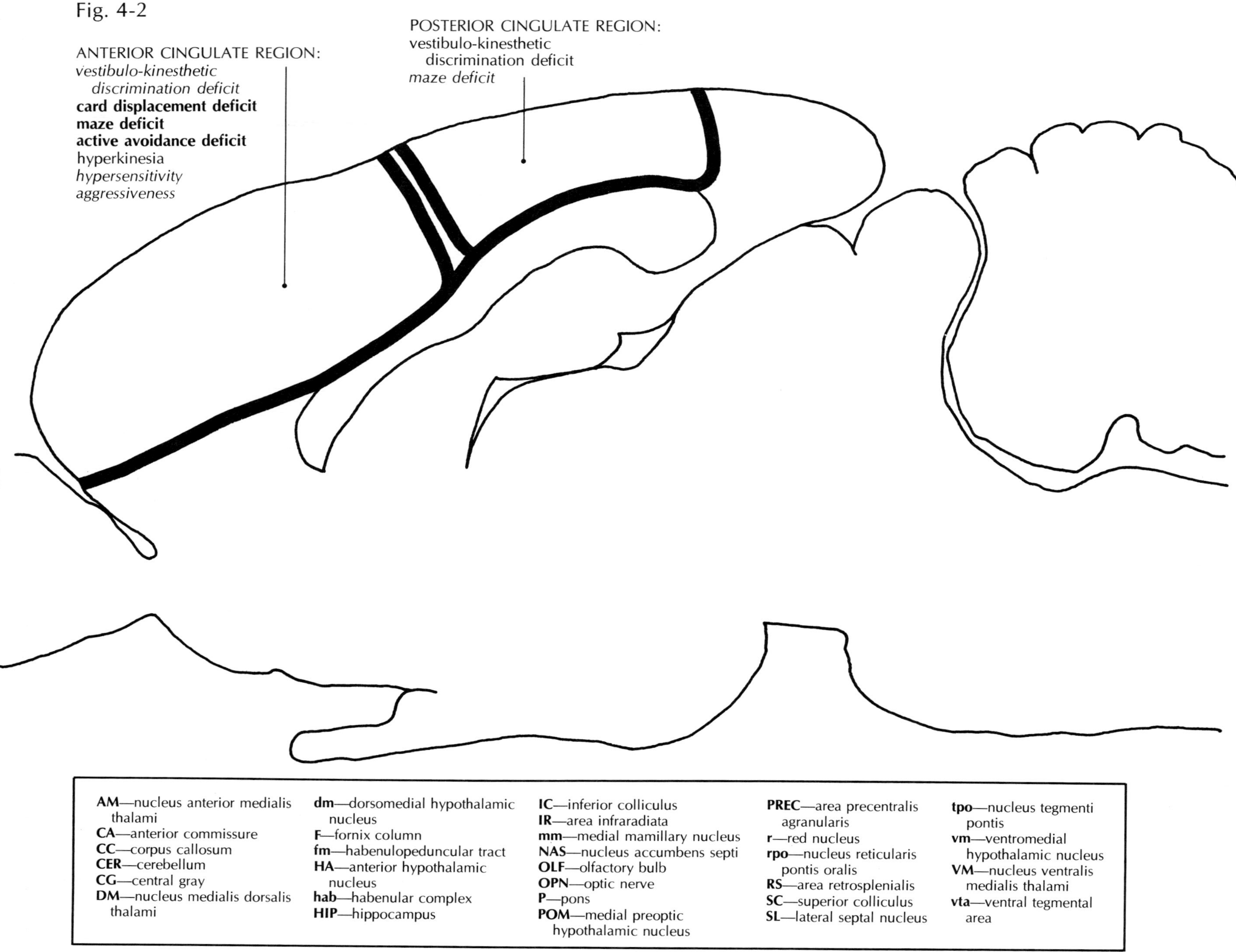

16

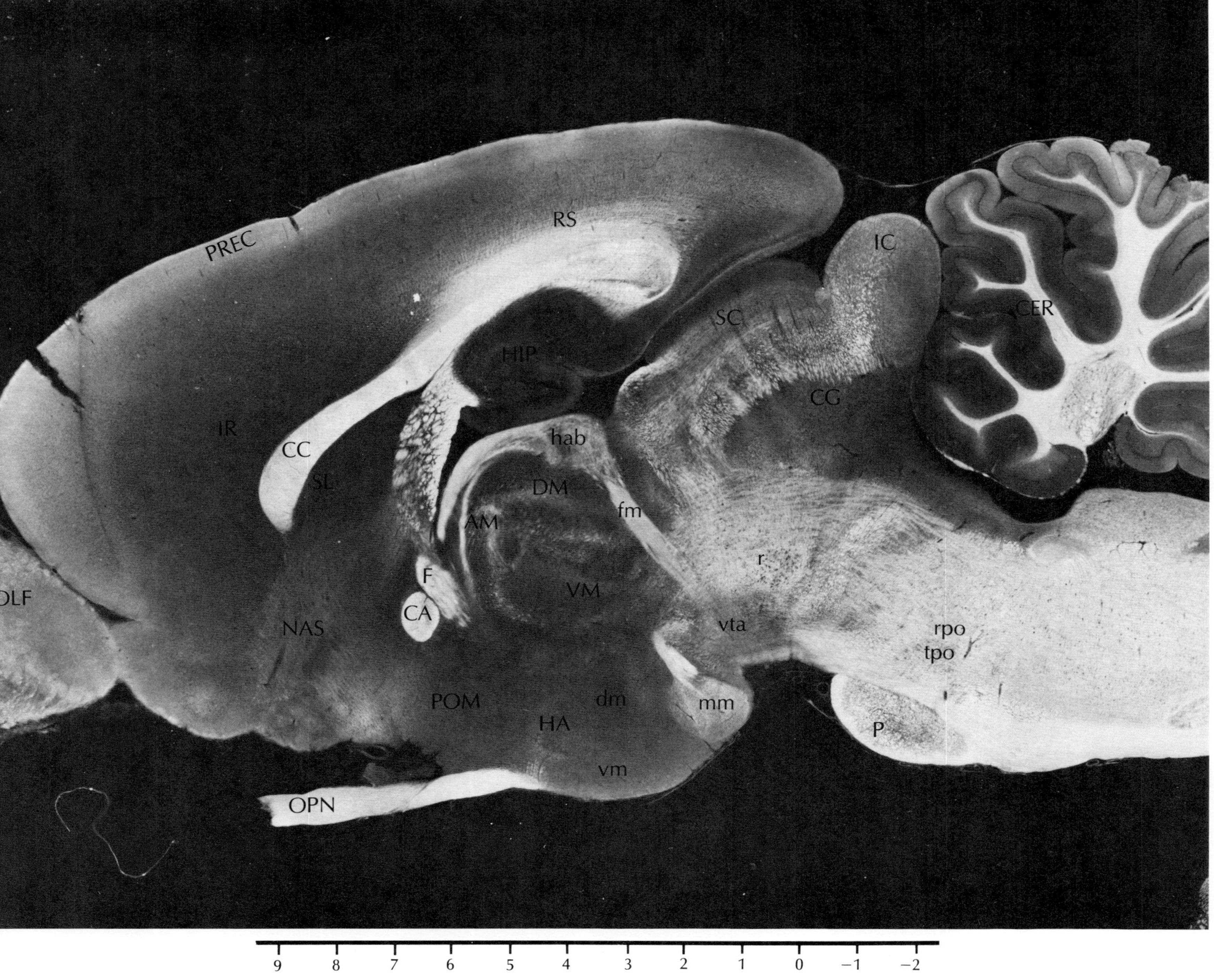

PREC
RS
IC
CER
SC
HIP
CG
IR
CC
hab
SL
DM
fm
AM
r
F
VM
OLF
CA
NAS
vta
rpo
tpo
POM
dm
mm
HA
P
vm
OPN
9 8 7 6 5 4 3 2 1 0 −1 −2

Fig. 4-3

ROSTRAL CAUDOPUTAMEN:
card displacement deficit
active avoidance deficit
escape response deficit
hyperkinesia
hypersensitivity
aggressiveness

NUCLEUS ACCUMBENS SEPTI:
card displacement deficit
active avoidance deficit
hyperkinesia
aggressiveness

caa—anterior commissure, anterior limb
CAPU—caudoputamen
CC—corpus callosum
MFB—medial forebrain bundle
NAS—nucleus accumbens septi
PYC—pyriform cortex
SL—lateral septal nucleus
SM—medial septal nucleus
TD—diagonal band of Broca
TOF—olfactory tubercle
tol—lateral olfactory tract

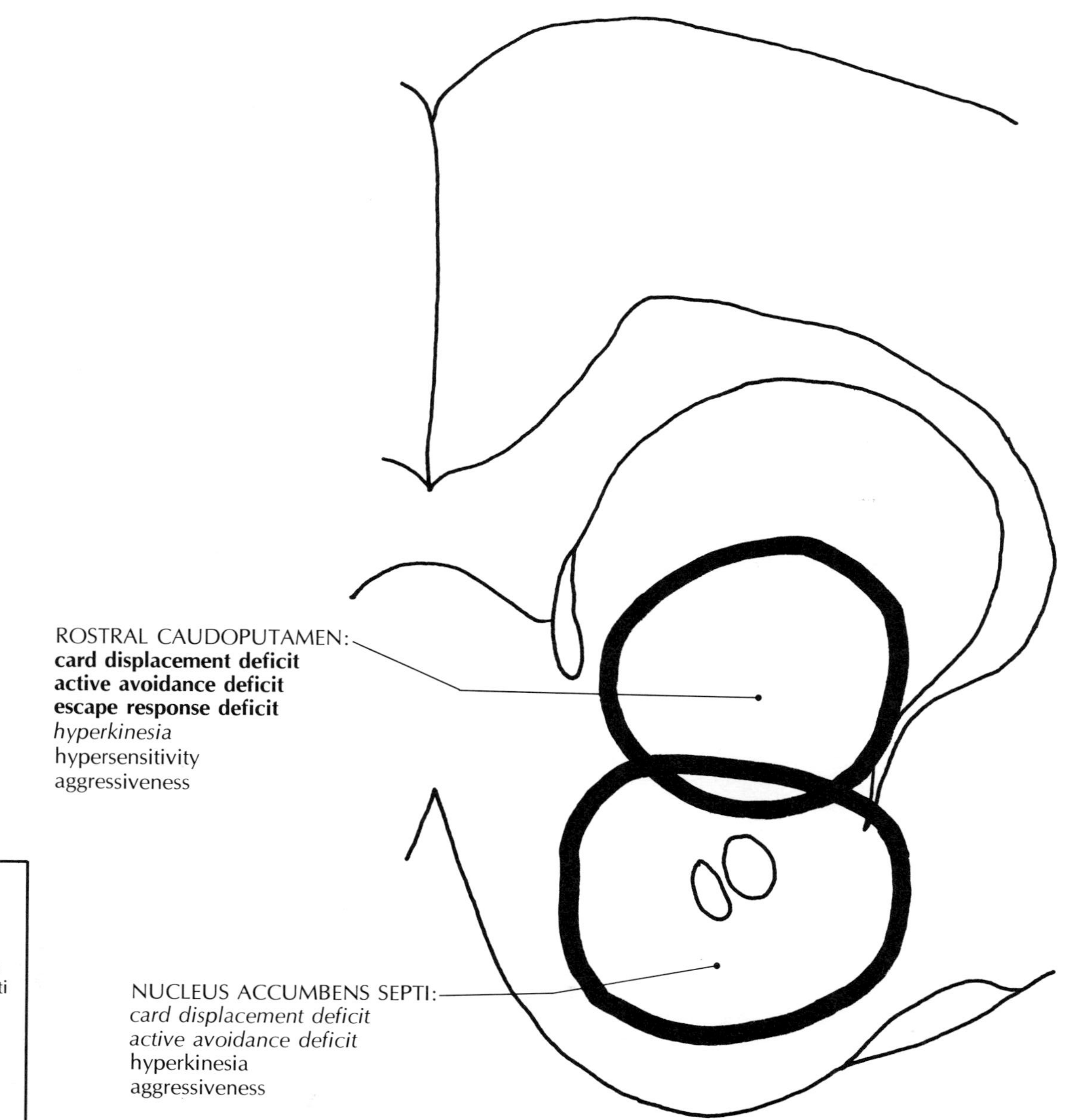

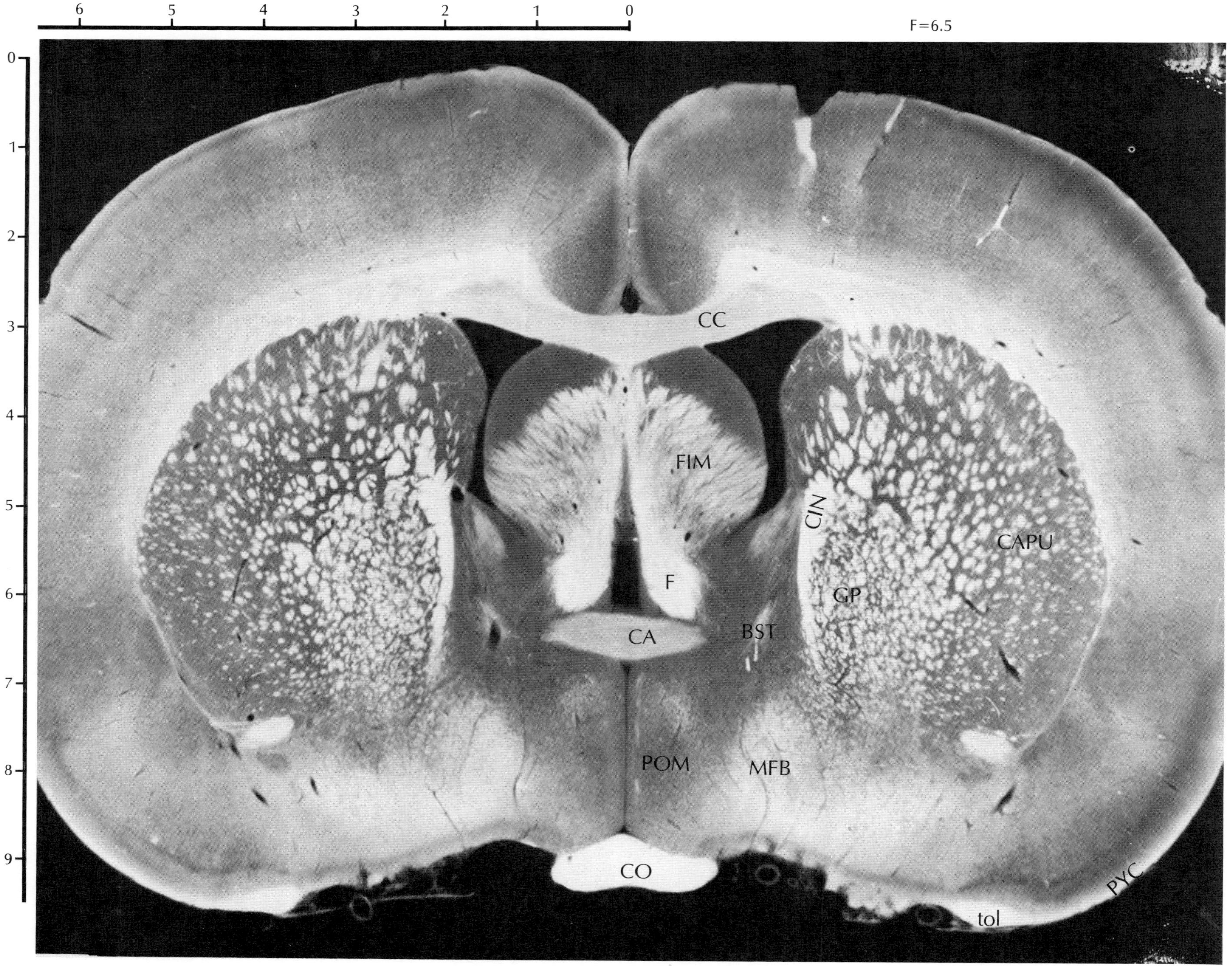

F=6.5
CC
FIM
CIN
CAPU
F
GP
CA
BST
POM
MFB
CO
tol
PYC

Fig. 4-6

ANTERIOR THALAMUS:
vestibulo-kinesthetic
    discrimination deficit
card displacement deficit
maze deficit
active avoidance deficit
escape response deficit
hypokinesia
hypersensitivity
aggressiveness

MEDIAL SUPRAOPTIC
HYPOTHALAMUS:
hypersensitivity
aggressiveness
high mortality rate

AM—nucleus anterior medialis
    thalami
AV—nucleus anterior ventralis
    thalami
CAPU—caudoputamen
CC—corpus callosum
CIN—internal capsule
CO—optic chiasma
F—fornix column
FIM—fimbria
GP—globus pallidus
HA—anterior hypothalamic
    nucleus
MFB—medial forebrain bundle
PT—nucleus paratenialis
PYC—pyriform cortex
R—nucleus reticularis
    thalami
RE—nucleus reuniens
sm—stria medullaris

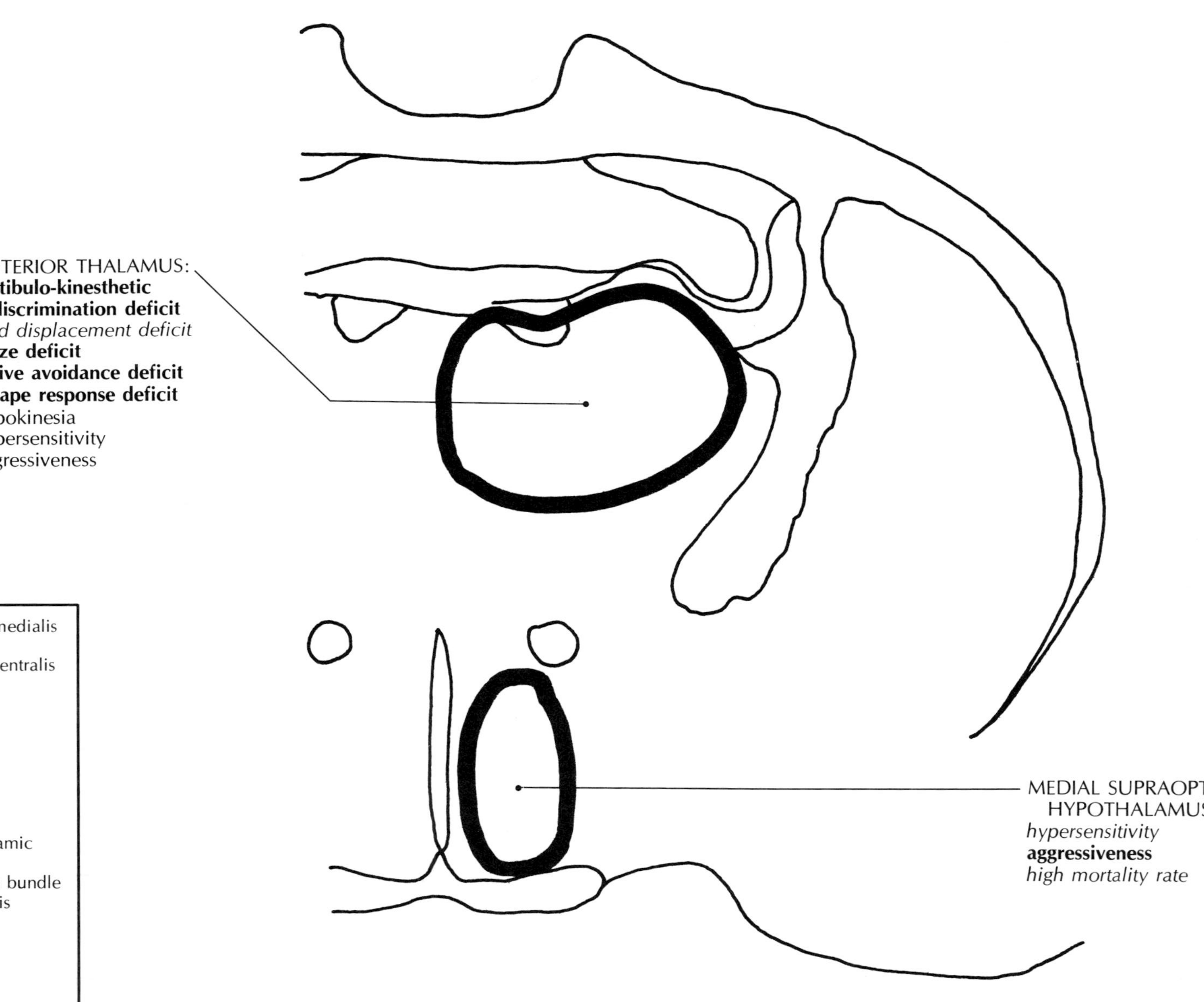

24

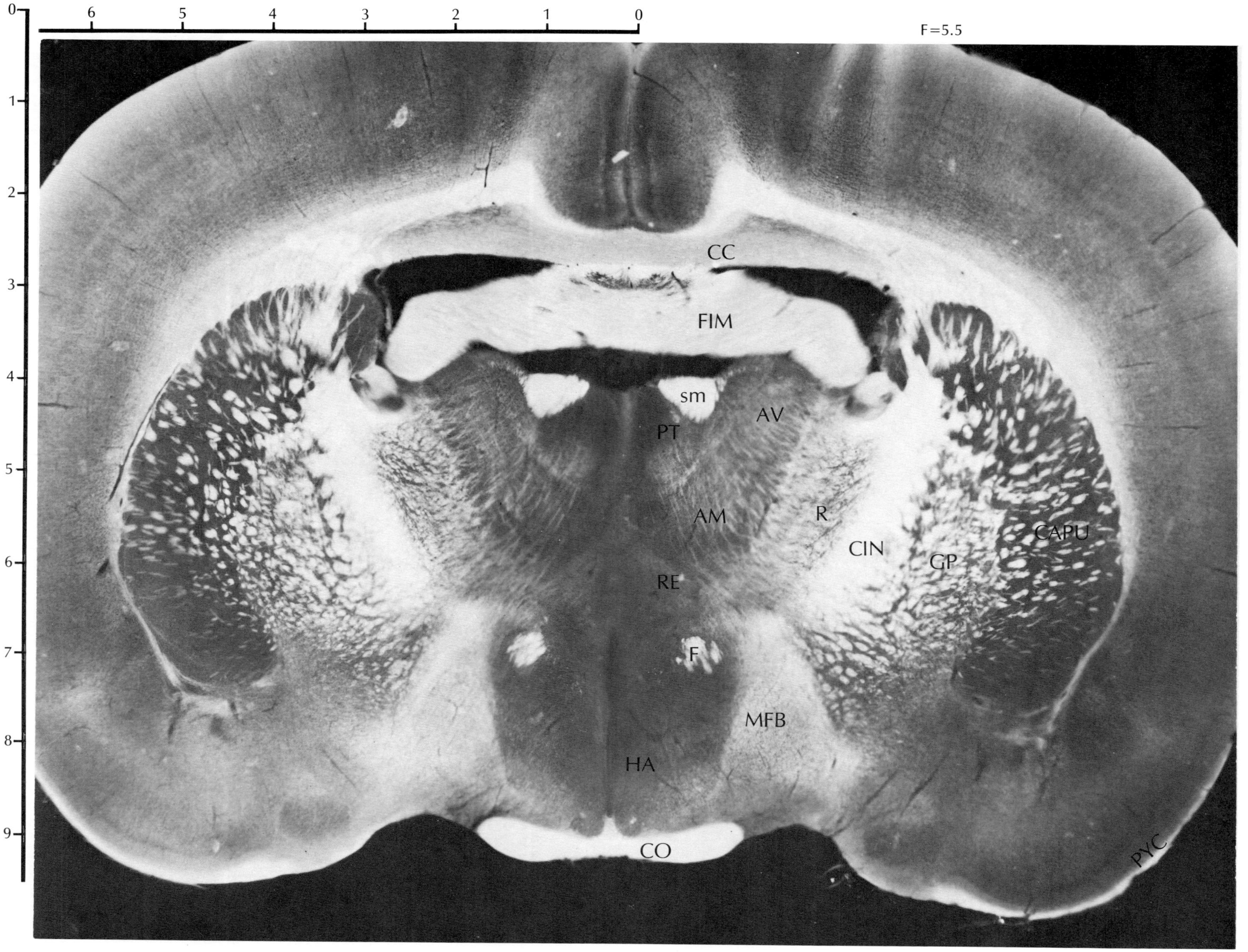

F=5.5
CC
FIM
sm
PT
AV
AM
R
CIN
GP
CAPU
RE
F
MFB
HA
CO
PYC

Fig. 4-7

aba—basal amygdaloid nucleus
aca—central amygdaloid nucleus
ala—lateral amygdaloid nucleus
ama—medial amygdaloid nucleus
CAPU—caudoputamen
CC—corpus callosum
CIN—internal capsule
coa—cortical amygdaloid nucleus
dm—dorsomedial hypothalamic nucleus
DM—nucleus medialis dorsalis thalami
EP—entopeduncular nucleus
F—fornix column
FIM—fimbria
GP—globus pallidus
hab—habenular complex
HIP—hippocampus
L—nucleus lateralis thalami
MFB—medial forebrain bundle
PYC—pyriform cortex
RE—nucleus reuniens
RH—nucleus rhomboideus
TO—optic tract
V—nucleus ventralis thalami
VD—nucleus ventralis thalami, pars dorsomedialis
vda—mamillothalamic tract
vm—ventromedial hypothalamic nucleus
VM—nucleus ventralis medialis thalami
ENTOPEDUNCULAR AREA:
visual discrimination deficit
vestibulo-kinesthetic discrimination deficit
card displacement deficit
maze deficit
active avoidance deficit
escape response deficit
obstinate progression
hypokinesia
hypersensitivity
aphagia-adipsia
AMYGDALA:
active avoidance deficit
escape response deficit
hypermetamorphosis
hyperkinesia

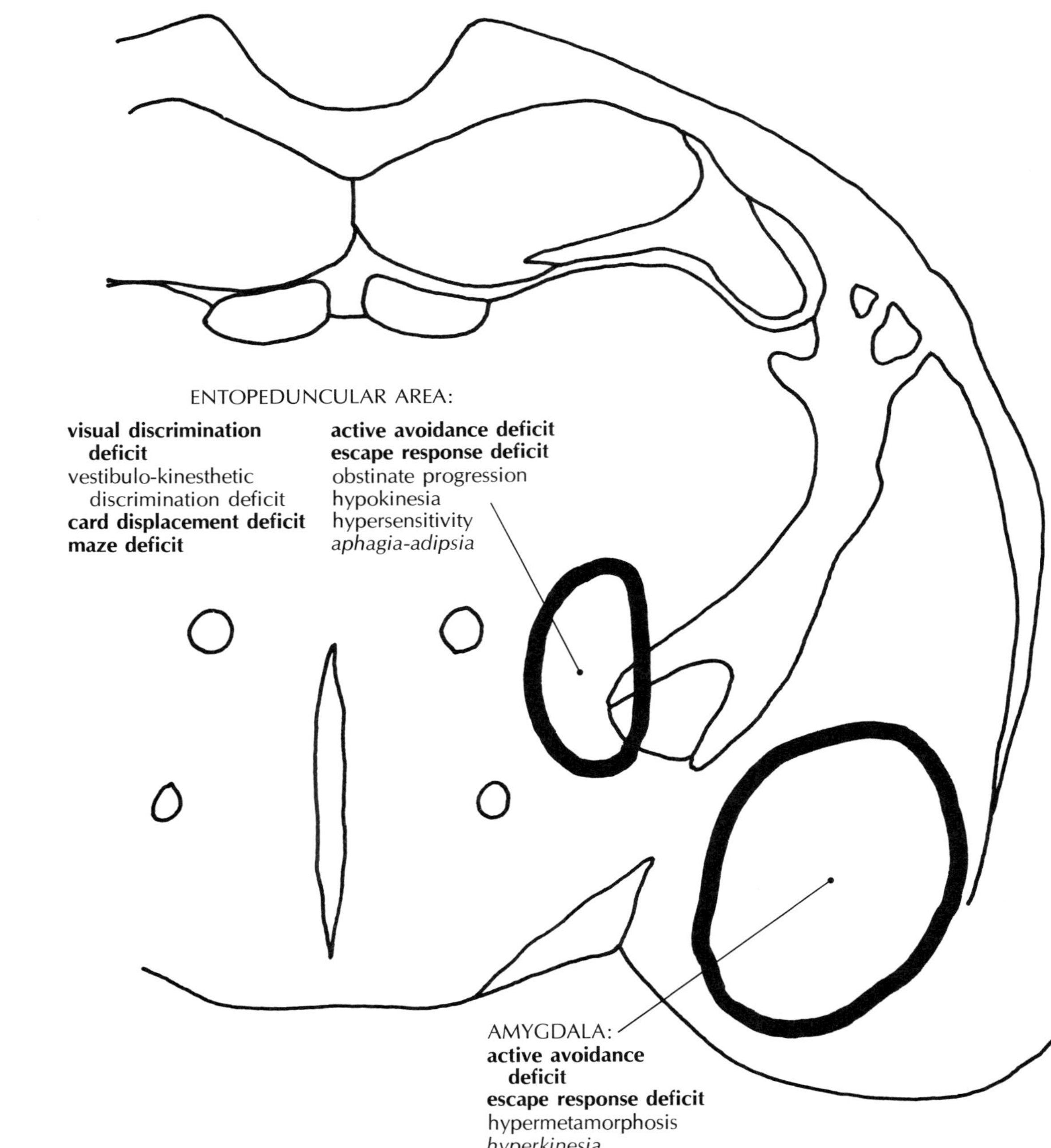

26

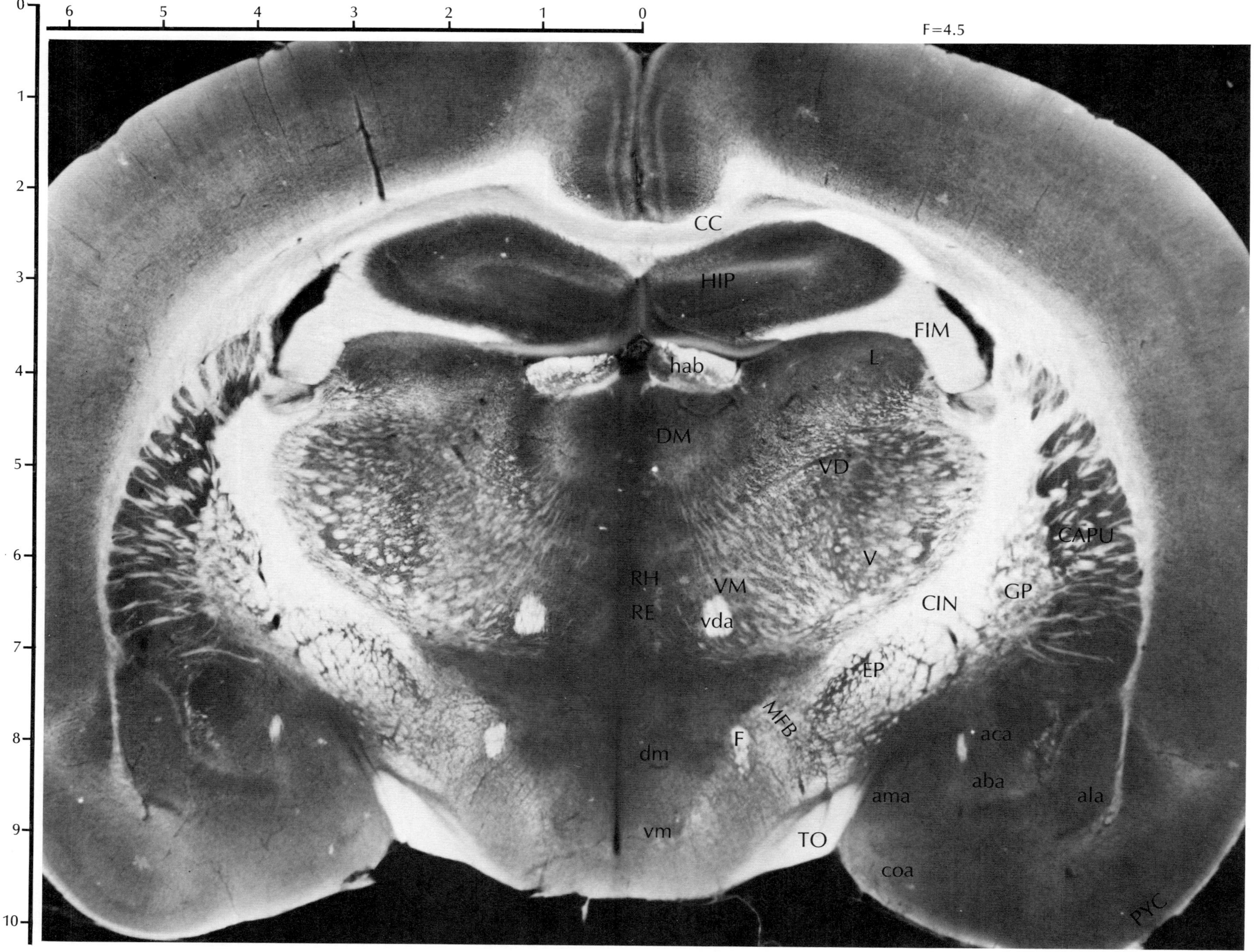

F=4.5
CC
HIP
FIM
L
hab
DM
VD
CAPU
V
RH
VM
CIN
GP
RE
vda
EP
MFB
F
aca
dm
aba
ama
ala
vm
TO
coa
PYC

Fig. 4-8

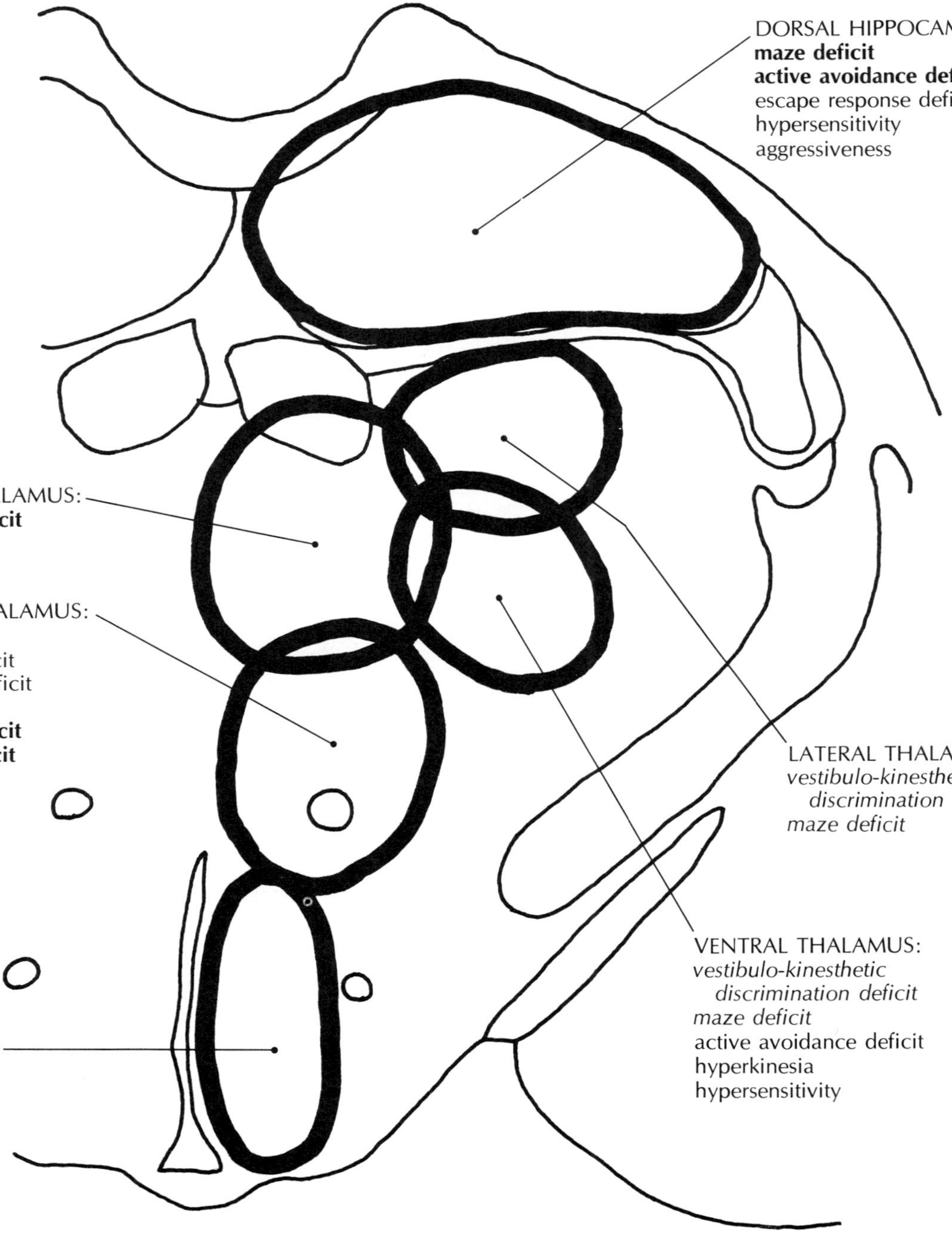

aba—basal amygdaloid nucleus
aca—central amygdaloid nucleus
ala—lateral amygdaloid nucleus
ama—medial amygdaloid nucleus
CAPU—caudoputamen
CC—corpus callosum
coa—cortical amygdaloid nucleus
dm—dorsomedial hypothalamic nucleus
F—fornix column
FIM—fimbria
GP—globus pallidus
hab—habenular complex
HIP—hippocampus
L—nucleus lateralis thalami
lm—medial lemniscus
MFB—medial forebrain bundle
mi—massa intermedia
PF—nucleus parafascicularis
PM—nucleus posteromedianus thalami
PP—cerebral peduncle
RE—nucleus reuniens
RH—nucleus rhomboideus
TO—optic tract
V—nucleus ventralis thalami
VD—nucleus ventralis thalami, pars dorsomedialis
vda—mamillothalamic tract
vm—ventromedial hypothalamic nucleus
VM—nucleus ventralis medialis thalami
zi—zona incerta

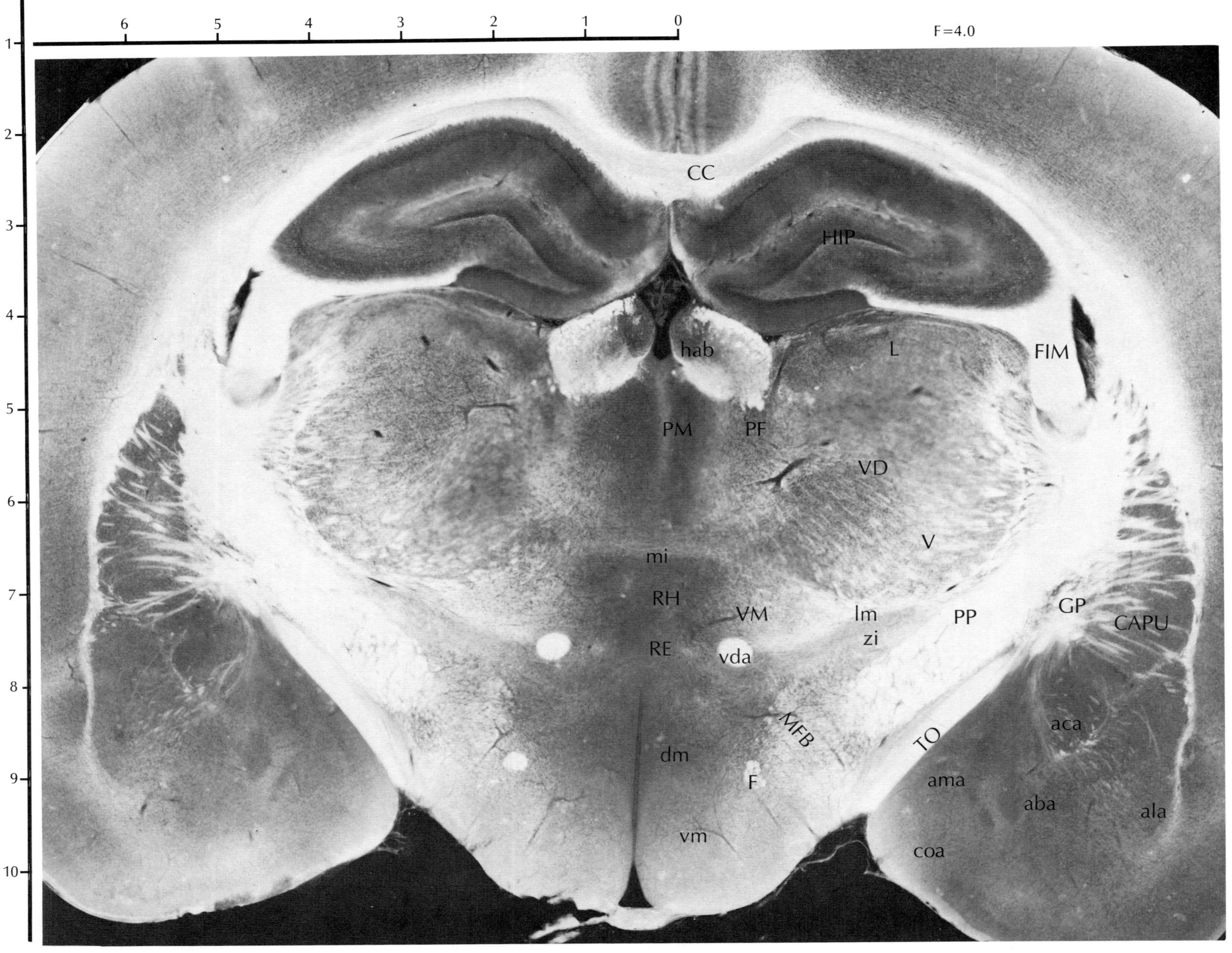

F=4.0
CC
HIP
hab
L
FIM
PM
PF
VD
V
mi
RH
VM
lm
zi
PP
GP
CAPU
RE
vda
MFB
TO
aca
dm
F
ama
aba
ala
vm
coa

Fig. 4-9

aba—basal amygdaloid nucleus
ala—lateral amygdaloid
  nucleus
CC—corpus callosum
coa—cortical amygdaloid
  nucleus
cs—subthalamic nucleus
dm—dorsomedial hypothalamic
  nucleus
ENT—entorhinal cortex
F—fornix column
fm—habenulopeduncular
  tract
GLD—lateral geniculate
  nucleus, pars dorsalis
GLV—lateral geniculate
  nucleus, pars ventralis
H₁—Forel's field H₁
H₂—Forel's field H₂
HIP—hippocampus
hp—posterior hypothalamic
  nucleus
lm—medial lemniscus
LP—nucleus lateralis
  thalami, pars posterior
MFB—medial forebrain bundle
NP—nucleus posterior thalami
p—nucleus pretectalis
pc—posterior commissure
PF—nucleus parafascicularis
PP—cerebral peduncle
TO—optic tract
tom—nucleus of the optic
  tract
V—nucleus ventralis
  thalami
vda—mamillothalamic tract
vm—ventromedial
  hypothalamic nucleus
zi—zona incerta

PRETECTAL AREA:
visual discrimination deficit
vestibulo-kinesthetic discrimination deficit
maze deficit
active avoidance deficit
escape response deficit
hypokinesia
hyperextension of the head
defective pupilloconstrictor reflex

NUCLEUS POSTERIOR AREA:
visual discrimination deficit
vestibulo-kinesthetic
  discrimination deficit
maze deficit
active avoidance deficit
escape response deficit
obstinate progression
hypokinesia
aphagia-adipsia

LATERAL GENICULATE NUCLEI:
visual discrimination deficit
maze deficit
hyperkinesia
hypersensitivity
aggressiveness
defective pupilloconstrictor
  reflex

PARAFASCICULAR AREA:
visual discrimination deficit
vestibulo-kinesthetic
  discrimination deficit
maze deficit
active avoidance deficit
escape response deficit
hypokinesia
hyperextension of the head

CAUDAL MEDIAL FOREBRAIN BUNDLE:
visual discrimination deficit
vestibulo-kinesthetic
  discrimination deficit
card displacement deficit
maze deficit
active avoidance deficit
escape response deficit
obstinate progression
hypokinesia
hypersensitivity
aphagia-adipsia
aggressiveness
somnolence
defective labyrinthine reflex

SUBTHALAMUS:
visual discrimination deficit
vestibulo-kinesthetic
  discrimination deficit
card displacement deficit
maze deficit
active avoidance deficit
escape response deficit
hypermetamorphosis
hypersensitivity
aphagia-adipsia

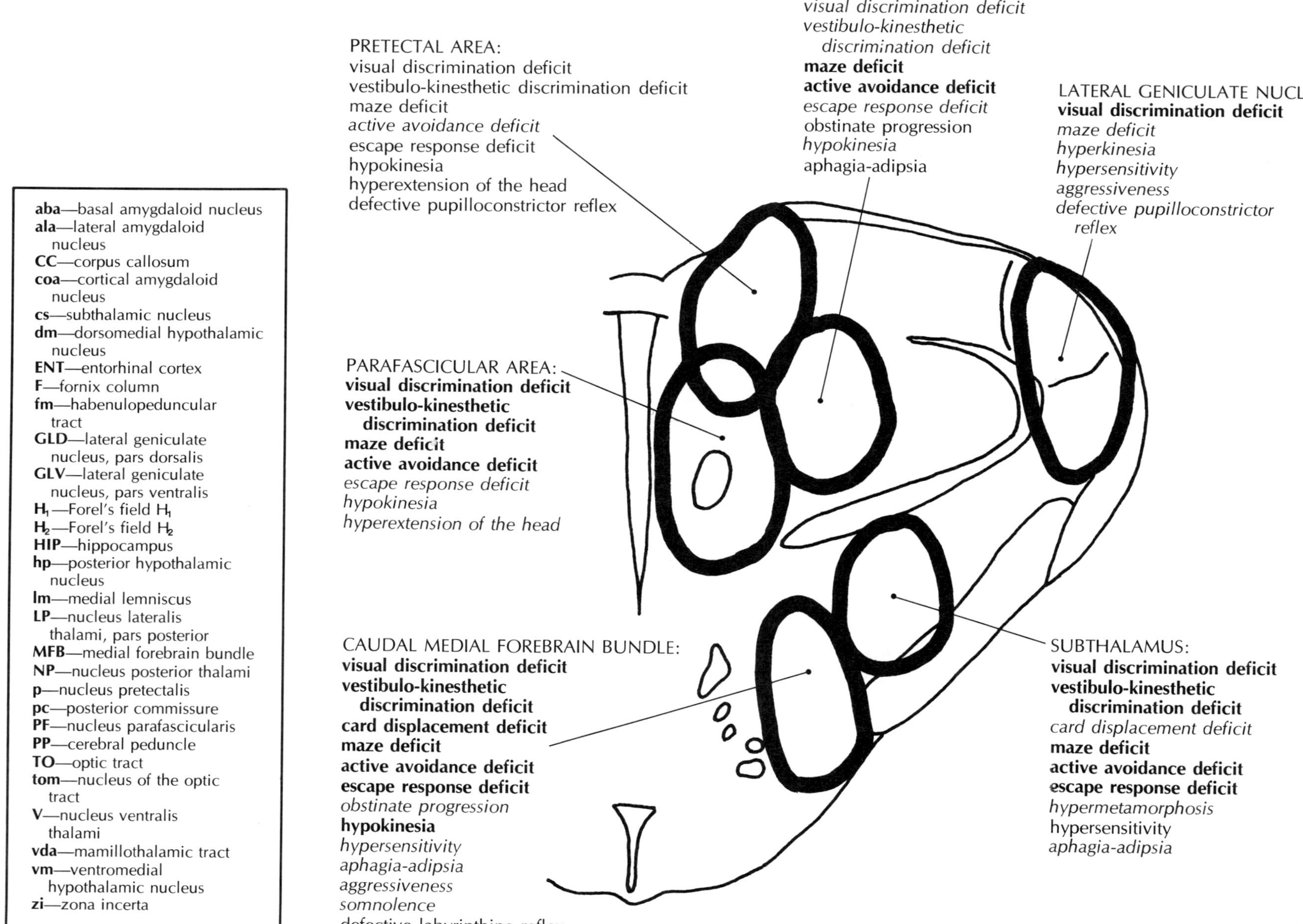

30

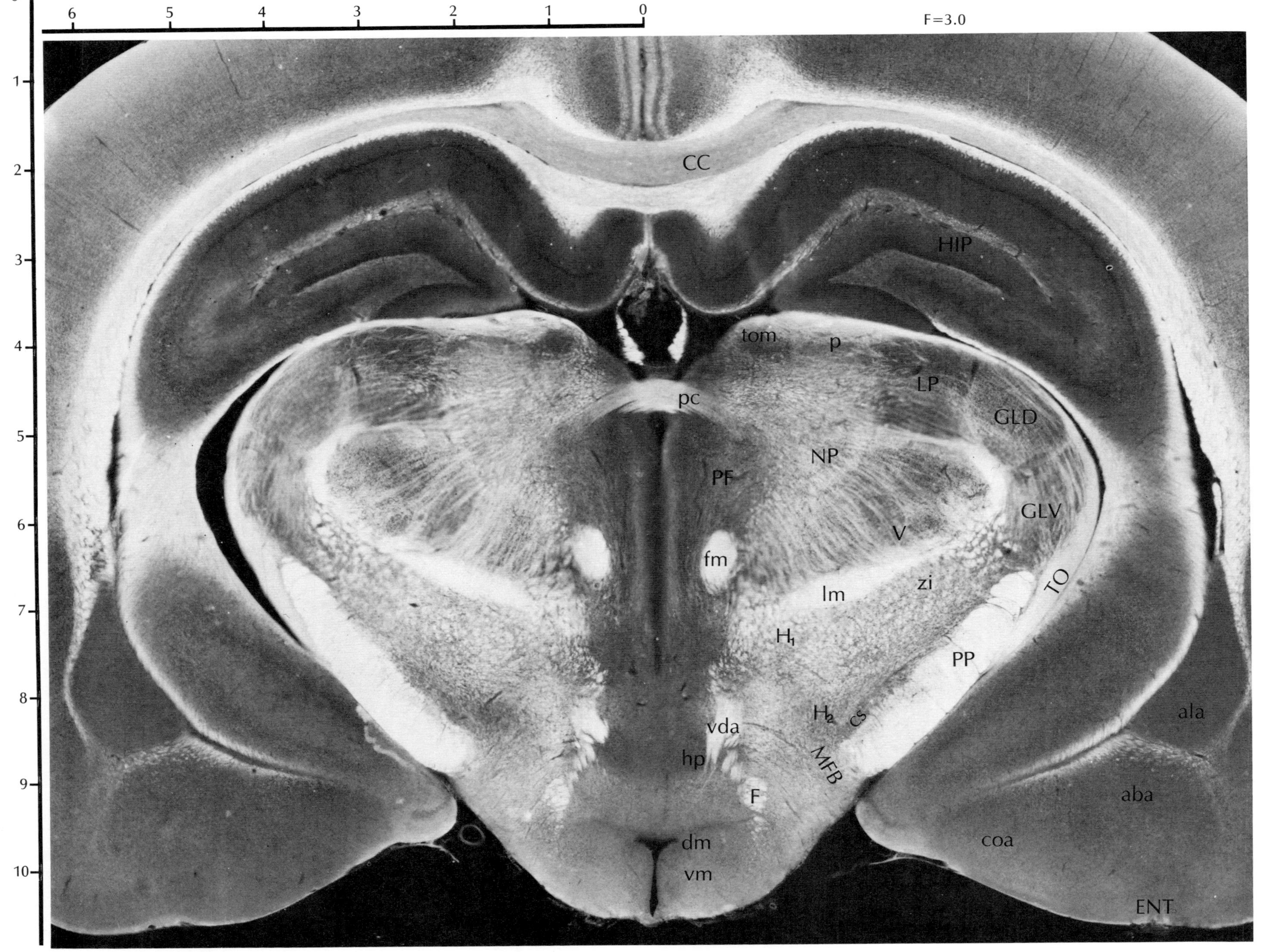

F=3.0
CC
HIP
tom
p
pc
LP
GLD
NP
PF
GLV
V
fm
zi
TO
lm
H1
PP
H2
cs
ala
vda
MFB
hp
F
aba
dm
coa
vm
ENT

Fig. 4-10

MEDIAL MESODIENCEPHALIC
RETICULAR FORMATION:
visual discrimination deficit
vestibulo-kinesthetic
discrimination deficit
maze deficit
active avoidance deficit
escape response deficit
aphagia-adipsia
hyperextension of the head
defective labyrinthine reflex

MAMILLARY BODIES:
card displacement deficit
maze deficit
active avoidance deficit
hypokinesia
hypersensitivity
hyperphagia

ala—lateral amygdaloid
nucleus
coa—cortical amygdaloid
nucleus
d—nucleus Darkschewitsch
ENT—entorhinal cortex
fm—habenulopeduncular
tract
GLD—lateral geniculate
nucleus, pars dorsalis
GLV—lateral geniculate
nucleus, pars ventralis
H₁—Forel's field H₁
H₂—Forel's field H₂
HIP—hippocampus
i—interstitial nucleus
of Cajal
LP—nucleus lateralis
thalami, pars posterior
lm—medial lemniscus
MFB—medial forebrain bundle
MG—medial geniculate
nucleus
ml—lateral mamillary
nucleus
mm—medial mamillary nucleus
NP—nucleus posterior
thalami
pc—posterior commissure
PP—cerebral peduncle
SC—superior colliculus
SNR—substantia nigra,
pars reticulata
sum—supramamillary
nucleus
zi—zona incerta

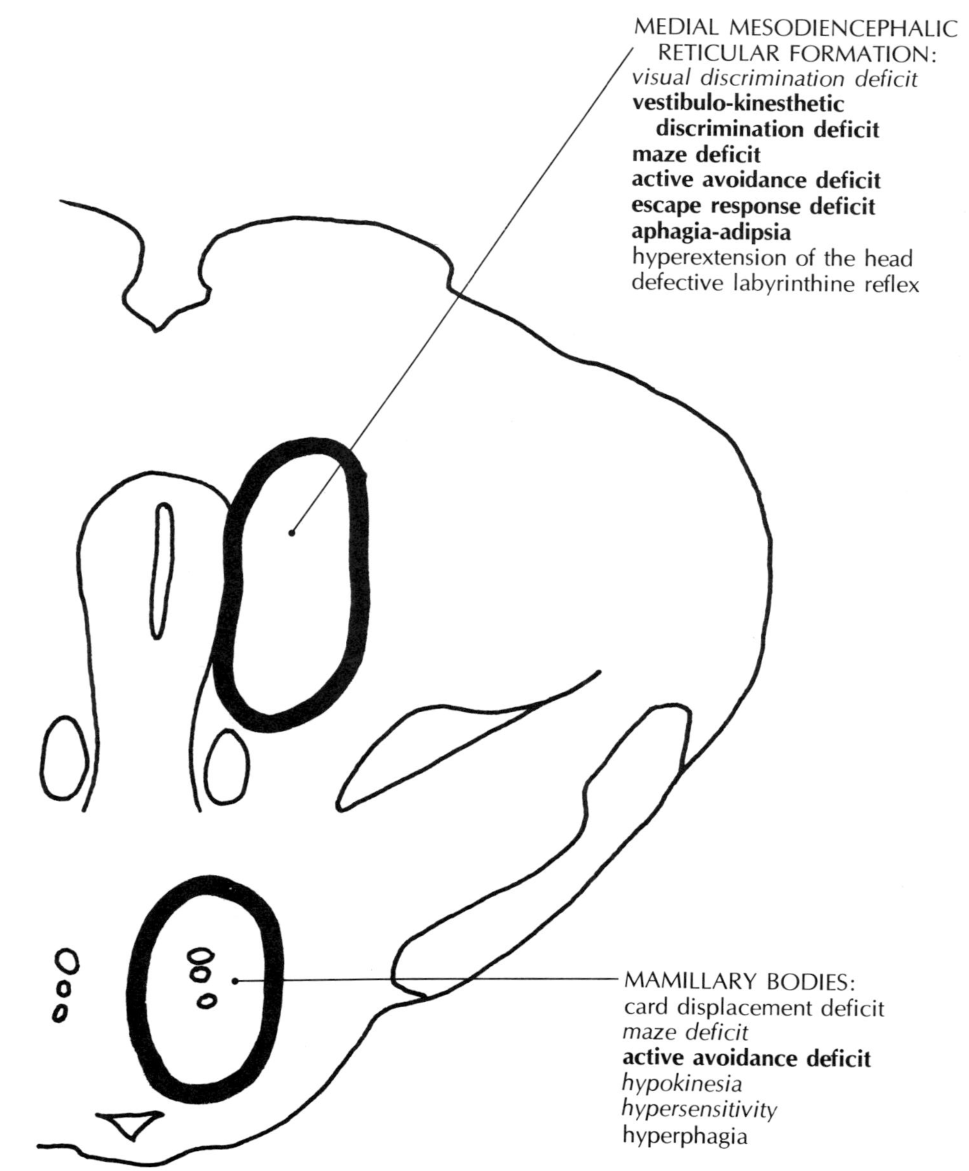

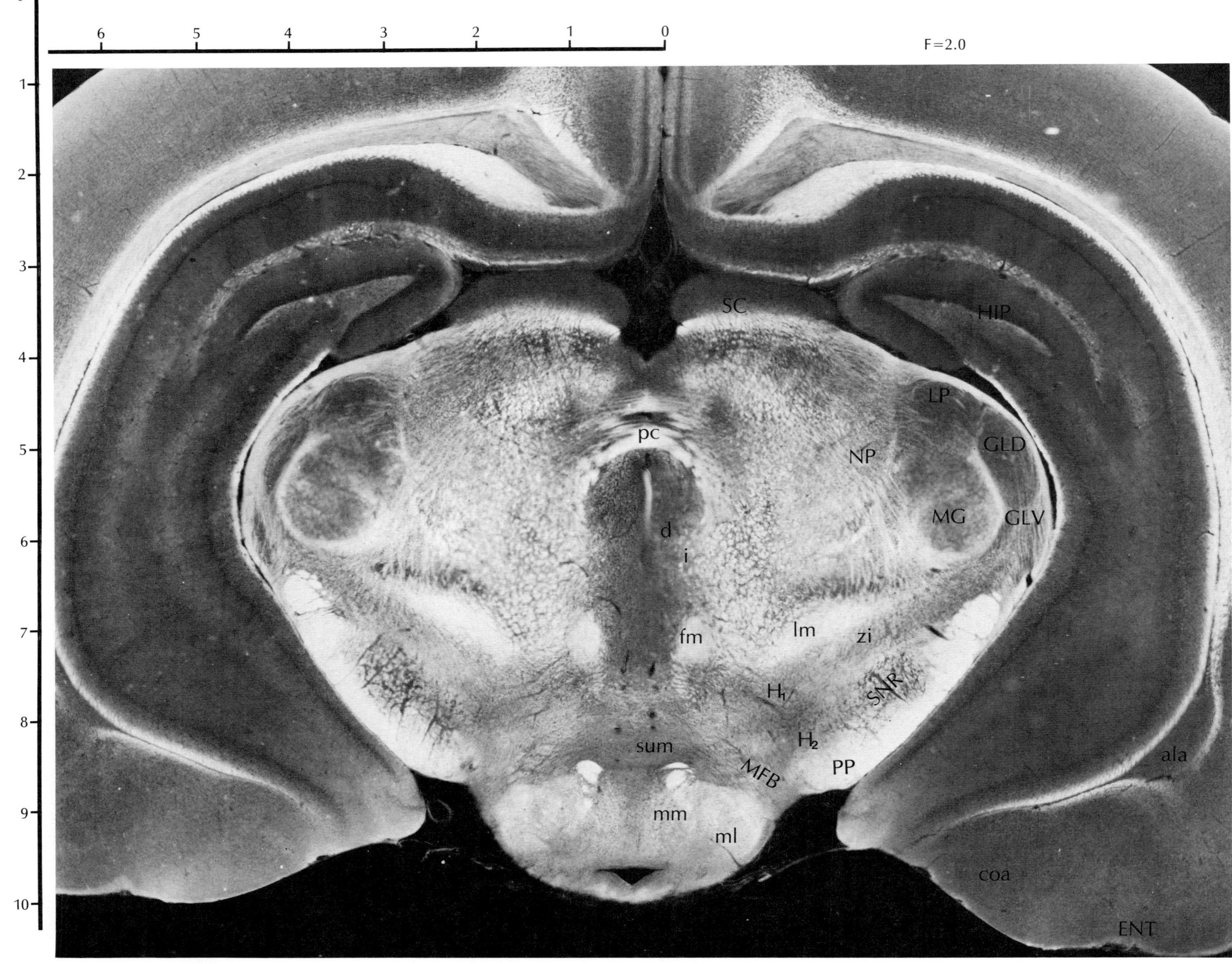

F=2.0
SC
HIP
LP
pc
NP
GLD
d
MG
GLV
i
lm
zi
fm
SNR
H₁
H₂
sum
PP
MFB
ala
mm
ml
coa
ENT

Fig. 4-11

SUPERIOR COLLICULUS:
active avoidance deficit
escape response deficit
hyperkinesia
hyperextension of the head

LATERAL PEDUNCULO-NIGRAL AREA:
visual discrimination deficit
card displacement deficit
maze deficit
active avoidance deficit
escape response deficit
hypermetamorphosis
hyperkinesia
hypersensitivity
aphagia-adipsia

PRERUBRAL AREA:
visual discrimination deficit
vestibulo-kinesthetic
   discrimination deficit
maze deficit
active avoidance deficit
escape response deficit
hypokinesia
aphagia-adipsia
abnormality of gait
defective labyrinthine reflex

VENTRAL TEGMENTAL AREA:
visual discrimination
   deficit
vestibulo-kinesthetic
   discrimination deficit
card displacement deficit
maze deficit
active avoidance deficit
escape response deficit
obstinate progression
hypokinesia
aphagia-adipsia
abnormality of gait
somnolence
defective labyrinthine
   reflex

CCS—commissure of the
   superior colliculus
CG—central gray
d—nucleus Darkschewitsch
DTV—ventral tegmental
   decussation
ENT—entorhinal cortex
fm—habenulopeduncular
   tract
HIP—hippocampus
i—interstitial nucleus
   of Cajal
lm—medial lemniscus
MG—medial geniculate
   nucleus
MRF—mesencephalic reticular
   formation
ON—oculomotor complex
PP—cerebral peduncle
r—red nucleus
SC—superior colliculus
SNC—substantia nigra,
   pars compacta
SNL—substantia nigra,
   pars lateralis
SNR—substantia nigra,
   pars reticulata
vta—ventral tegmental area

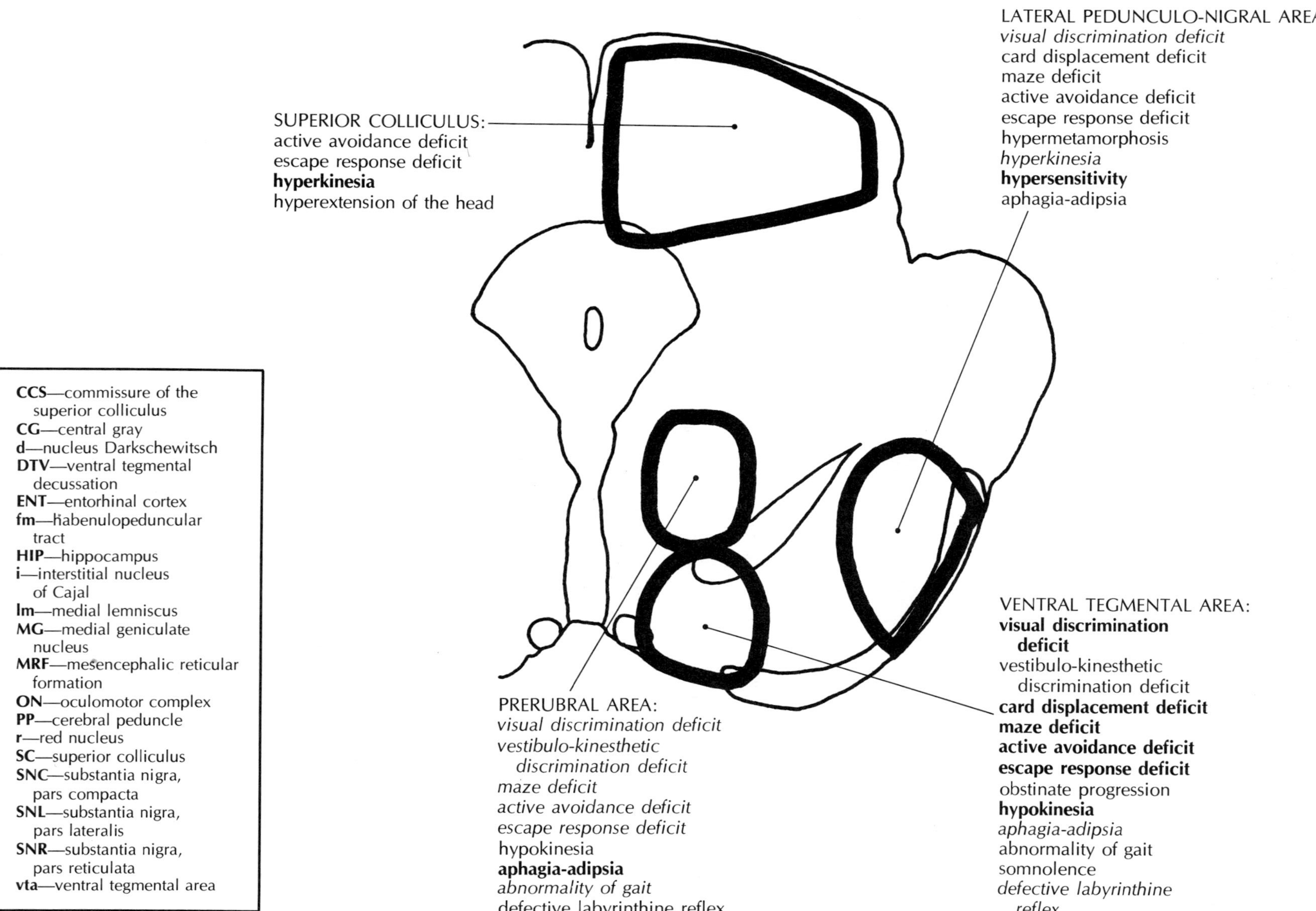

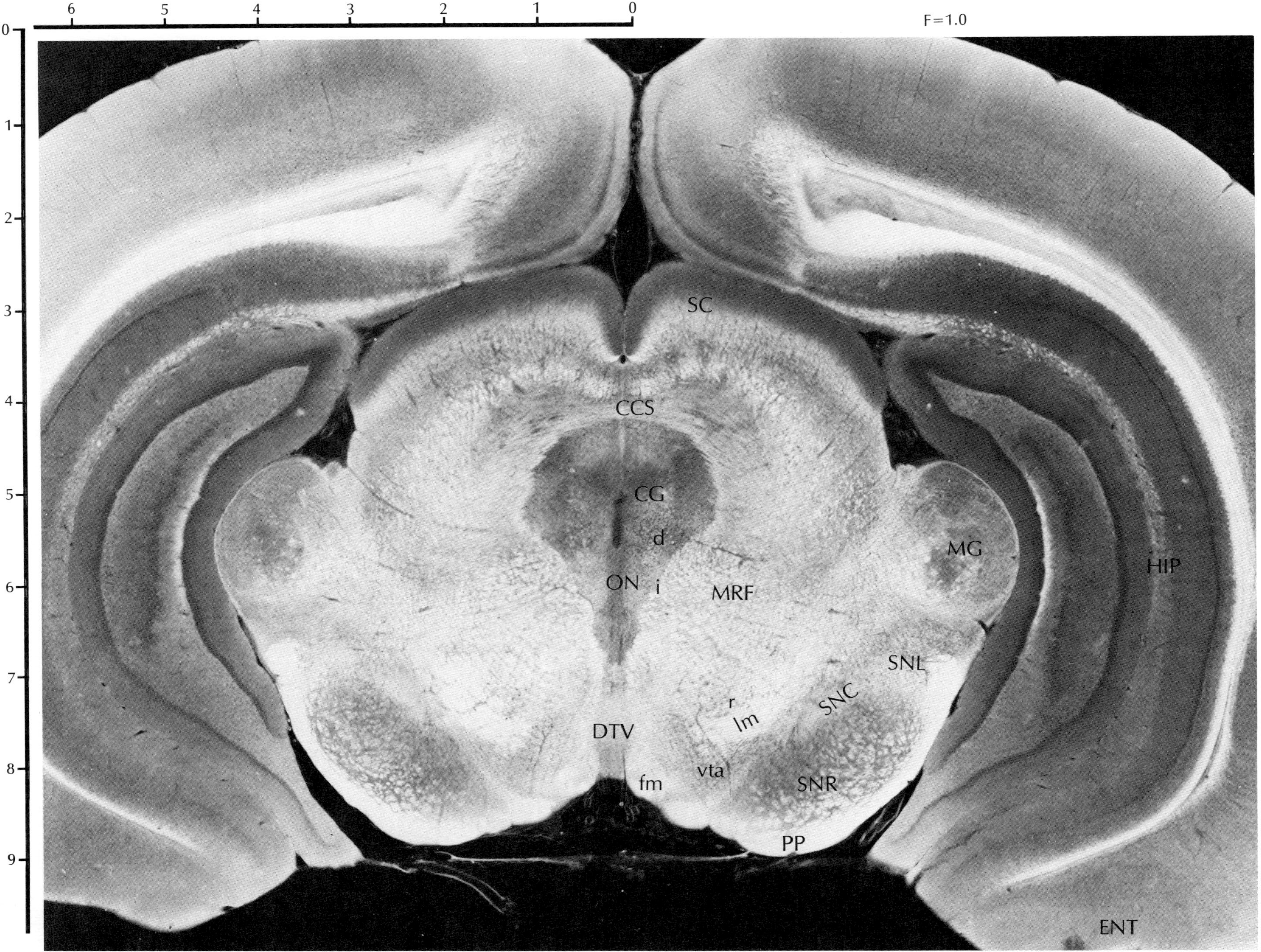

F=1.0
SC
CCS
CG
d
ON i
MRF
MG
HIP
SNL
r
lm
SNC
DTV
vta
SNR
fm
PP
ENT

Fig. 4-12

SUPRARUBRAL RETICULAR FORMATION:
vestibulo-kinesthetic
  discrimination deficit
active avoidance deficit
hyperkinesia
aphagia-adipsia
coma
defective labyrinthine
  reflex
high mortality rate

RED NUCLEUS AREA:
visual discrimination deficit
vestibulo-kinesthetic
  discrimination deficit
maze deficit
hyperkinesia
aphagia-adipsia
abnormality of gait
defective labyrinthine
  reflex
high mortality rate

SUBCOLLICULAR TEGMENTUM:
vestibulo-kinesthetic
  discrimination deficit
hyperkinesia
coma

SUPRANIGRAL RETICULAR
  FORMATION:
maze deficit
active avoidance deficit
escape response deficit
hyperkinesia
aphagia-adipsia
jerky head movements
hyperextension of the head

SUBSTANTIA NIGRA:
visual discrimination deficit
vestibulo-kinesthetic
  discrimination deficit
card displacement deficit
maze deficit
active avoidance deficit
escape response deficit
hypermetamorphosis
hyperkinesia
aphagia-adipsia
jerky head movements
abnormality of gait

INTERPEDUNCULO-CENTRAL
TEGMENTAL AREA:
vestibulo-kinesthetic
  discrimination deficit
maze deficit
active avoidance deficit
escape response deficit
defective pupilloconstrictor
  reflex
defective labyrinthine reflex

CCS—commissure of the
  superior colliculus
CG—central gray
DTD—dorsal tegmental decussation
DTV—ventral tegmental decussation
HIP—hippocampus
ip—interpeduncular nucleus
lm—medial lemniscus
MG—medial geniculate
  nucleus
MRF—mesencephalic reticular
  formation
ON—oculomotor complex
PP—cerebral peduncle
r—red nucleus
SC—superior colliculus
SNC—substantia nigra,
  pars compacta
SNL—substantia nigra,
  pars lateralis
SNR—substantia nigra,
  pars reticulata
III—oculomotor nerve

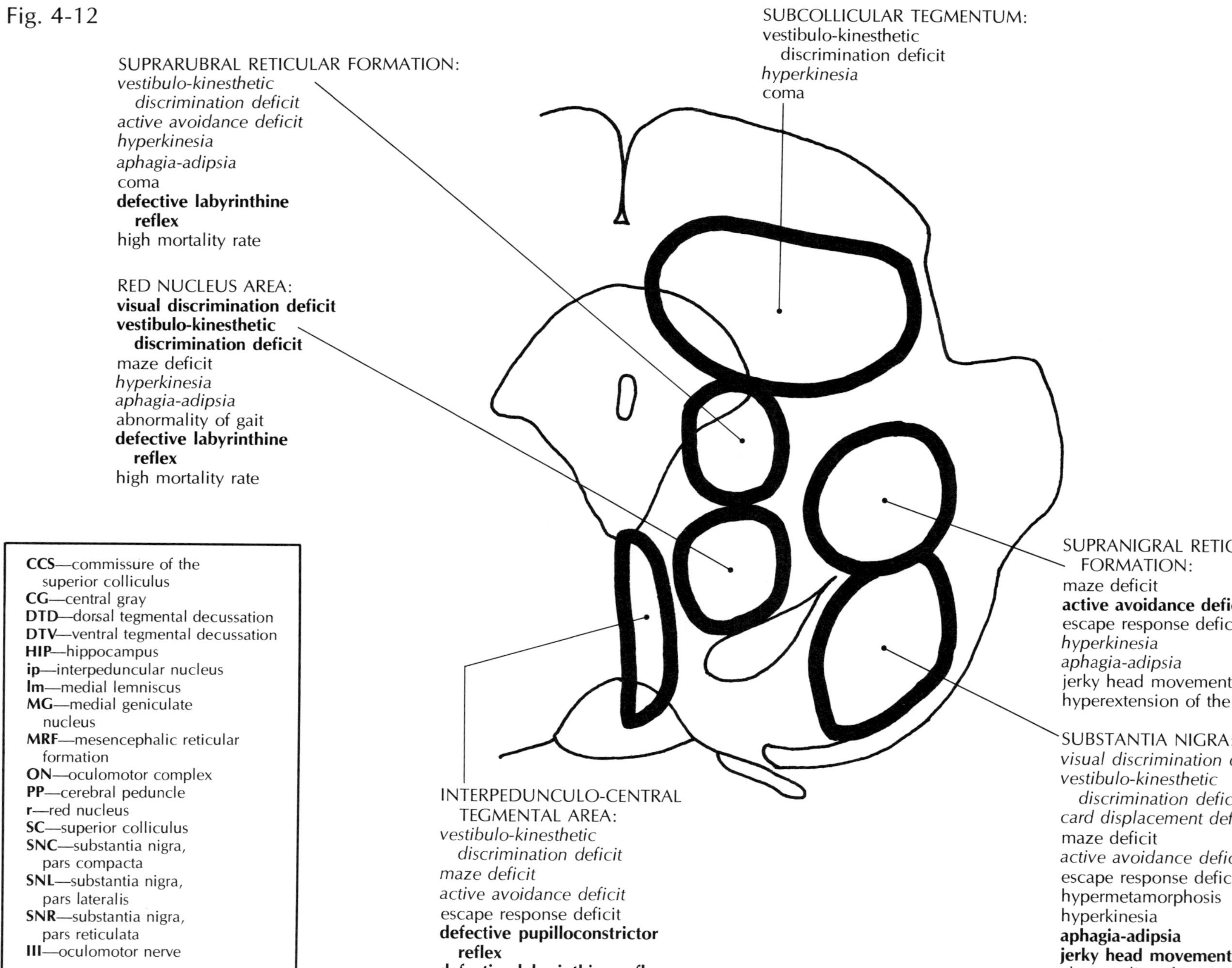

36

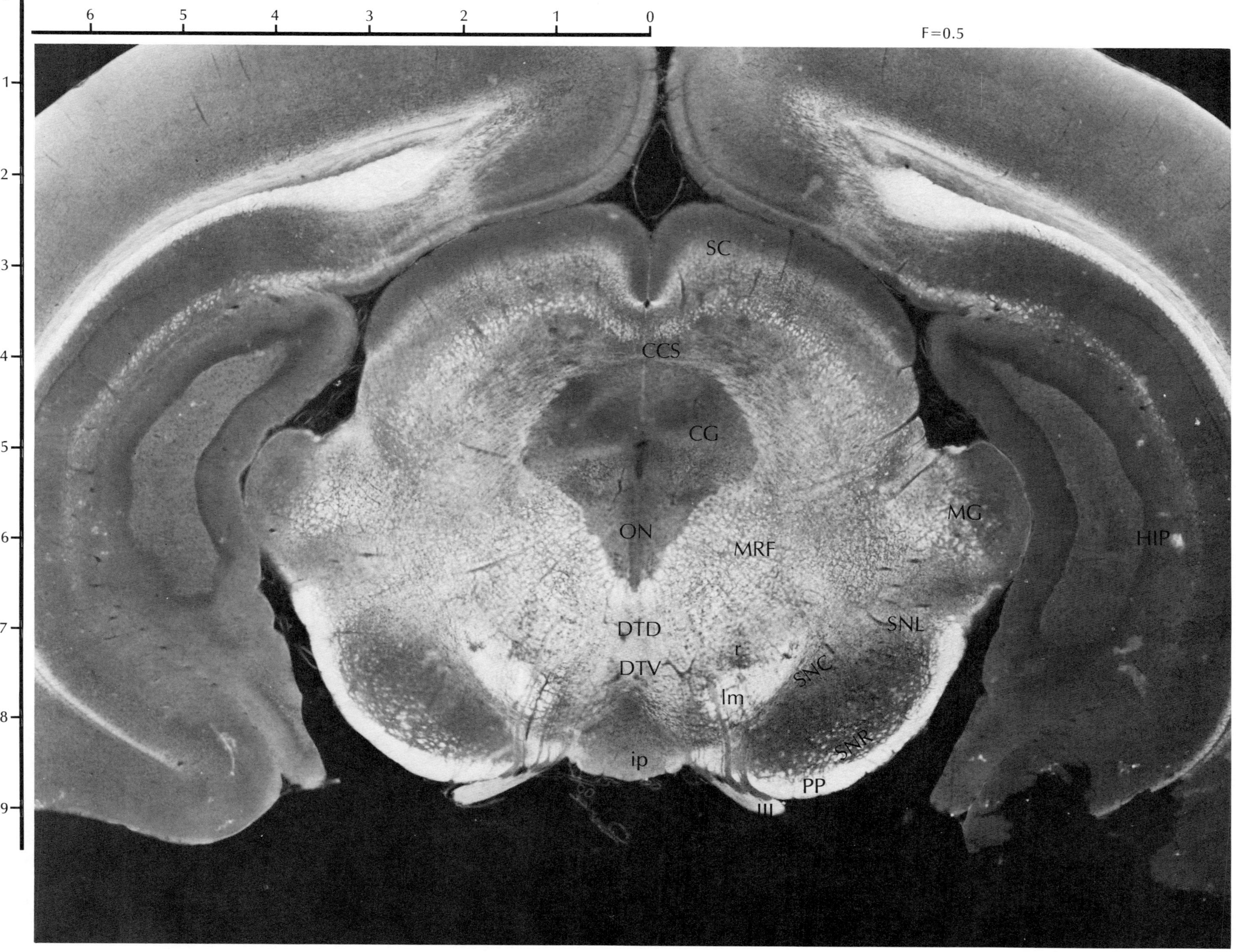

F=0.5
SC
CCS
CG
ON
MRF
MG
HIP
DTD
DTV
r
lm
SNL
SNC
SNR
PP
III
ip

Fig. 4-13

CENTRAL GRAY AREA:
vestibulo-kinesthetic
  discrimination deficit
escape response deficit
hyperkinesia
hyperphagia
coma
defective pupilloconstrictor
  reflex
defective labyrinthine reflex

POSTRUBRAL RETICULAR
  FORMATION:
visual discrimination deficit
vestibulo-kinesthetic
  discrimination deficit
maze deficit
active avoidance deficit
obstinate progression
hyperkinesia
aphagia-adipsia
abnormality of gait
defective labyrinthine reflex
high mortality rate

VENTROLATERAL MIDBRAIN
  RETICULAR FORMATION:
visual discrimination deficit
vestibulo-kinesthetic
  discrimination deficit
maze deficit
active avoidance deficit
escape response deficit
hyperkinesia
aphagia-adipsia
jerky head movements
abnormality of gait

CCS—commissure of the
  superior colliculus
CG—central gray
ENT—entorhinal cortex
HIP—hippocampus
ip—interpeduncular
  nucleus
lc—nucleus linearis,
  pars caudalis
lm—medial lemniscus
MRF—mesencephalic reticular
  formation
ON—oculomotor complex
P—pons
PP—cerebral peduncle
r—red nucleus
SC—superior colliculus
SNR—substantia nigra,
  pars reticulata

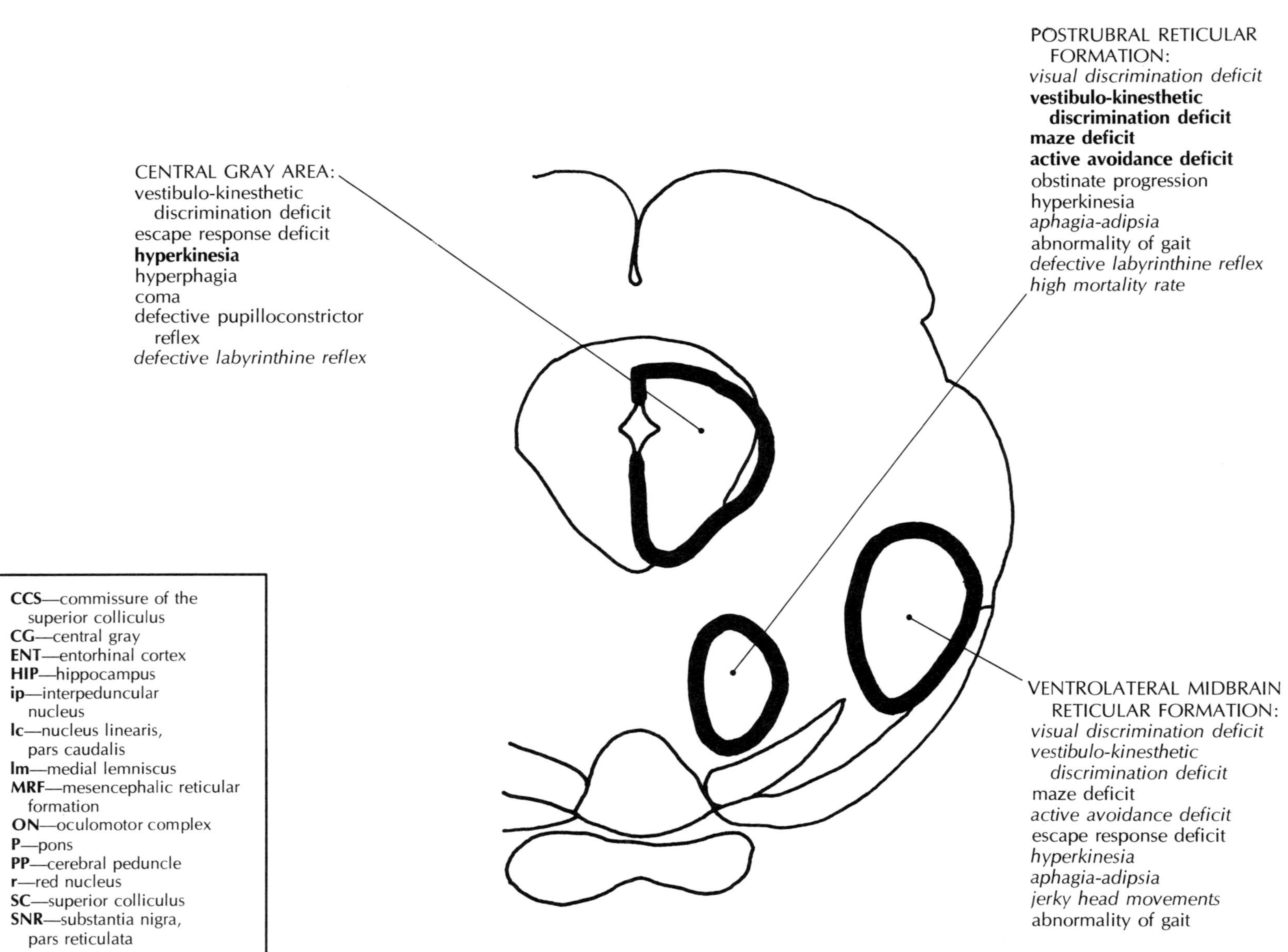

38

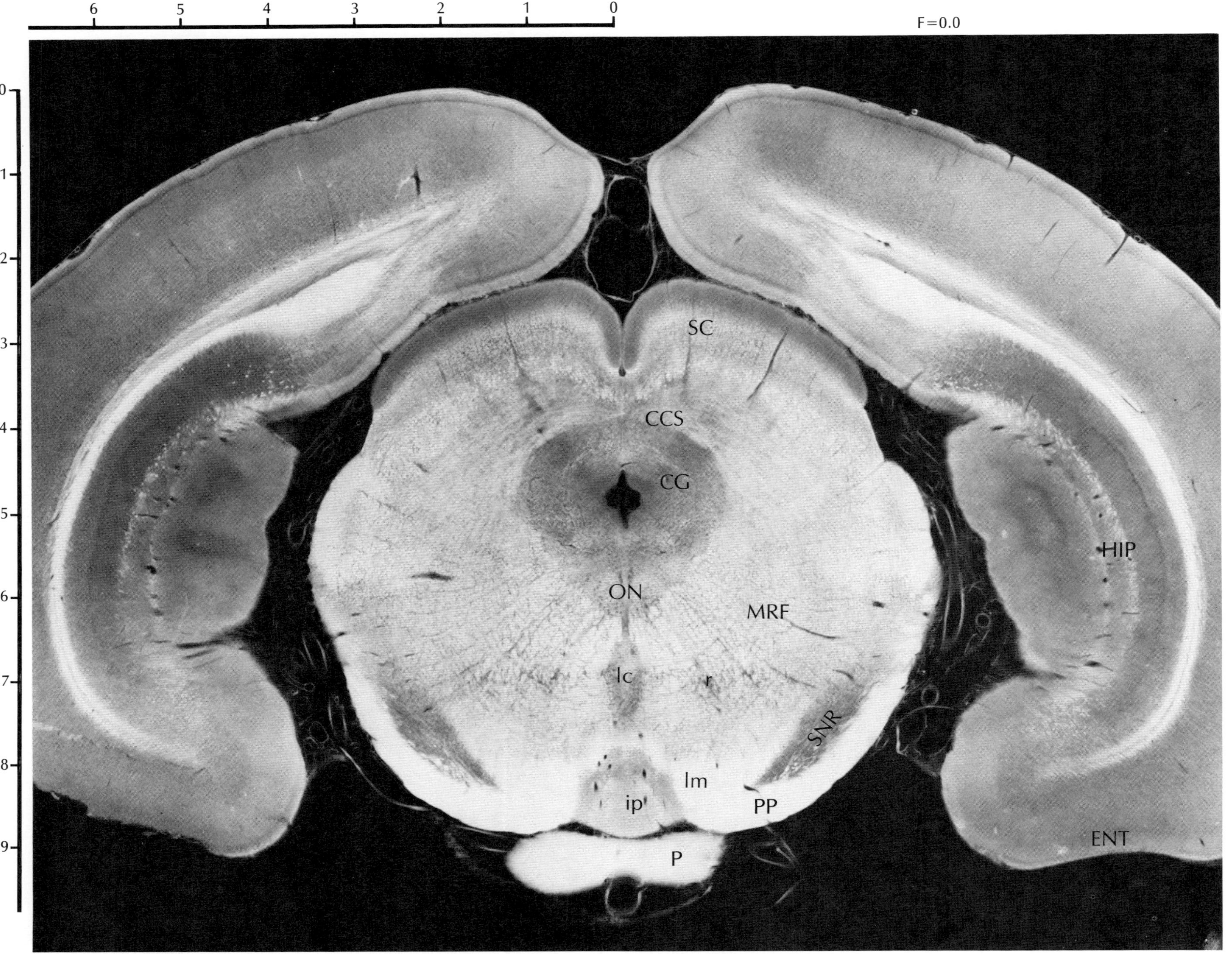

F=0.0
SC
CCS
CG
ON
MRF
SNR
HIP
Ic
lm
ip
PP
P
ENT

Fig. 4-14

ENTORHINO-SUBICULAR AREA:
visual discrimination deficit
vestibulo-kinesthetic
    discrimination deficit
card displacement deficit
maze deficit
active avoidance deficit
escape response deficit
hypermetamorphosis
hyperkinesia
hypersensitivity
aggressiveness

CCS—commissure of the
    superior colliculus
CG—central gray
DBC—decussation of brachium
    conjunctivum
dr—nucleus dorsalis raphes
ENT—entorhinal cortex
IC—inferior colliculus
ip—interpeduncular nucleus
lc—nucleus linearis,
    pars caudalis
LL—lateral lemniscus
lm—medial lemniscus
MRF—mesencephalic reticular
    formation
ON—oculomotor complex
P—pons
pi—pineal body
PP—cerebral peduncle
SC—superior colliculus
SUB—subiculum
vrl—nucleus ventralis
    rostralis lemnisci
    lateralis

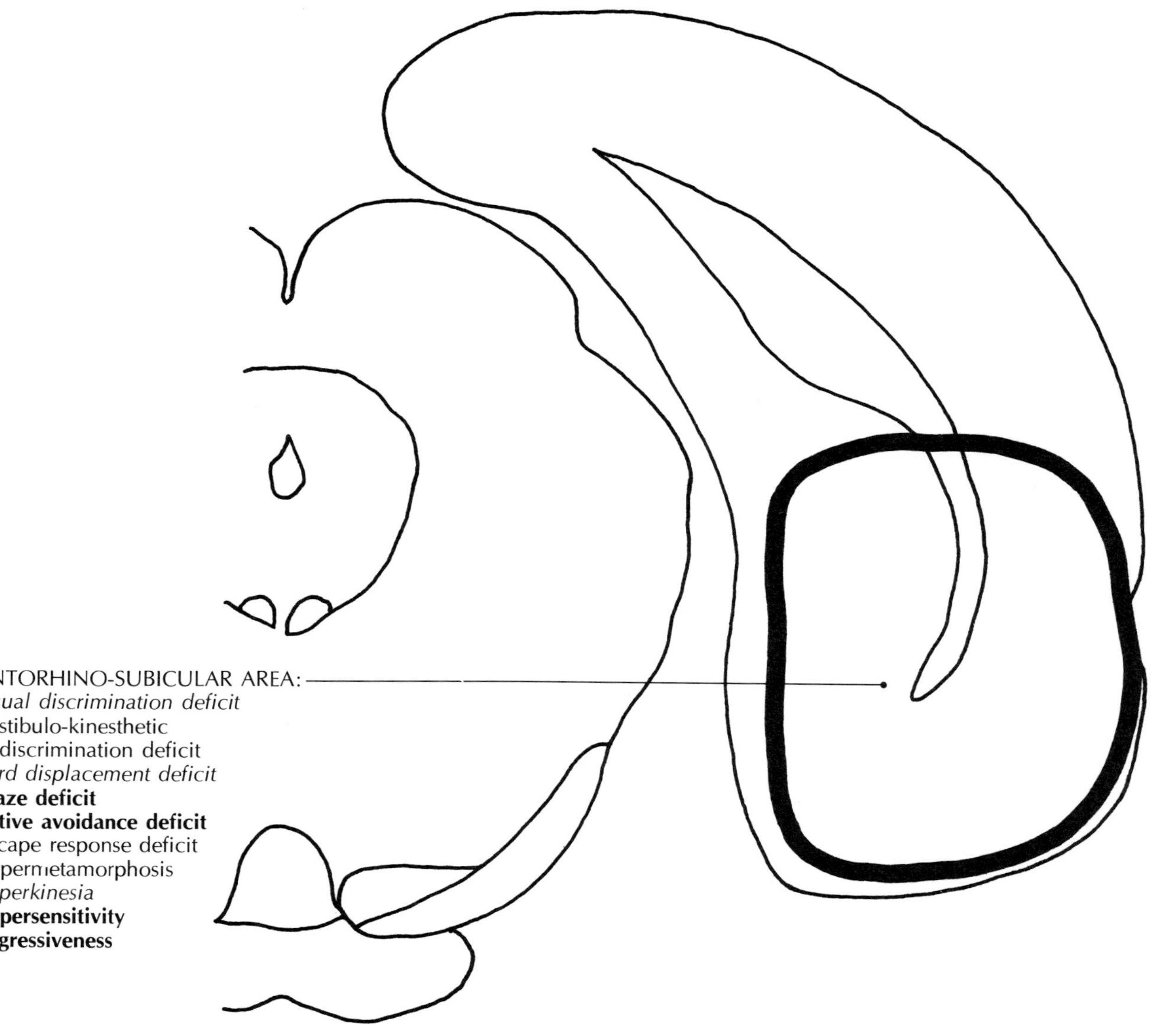

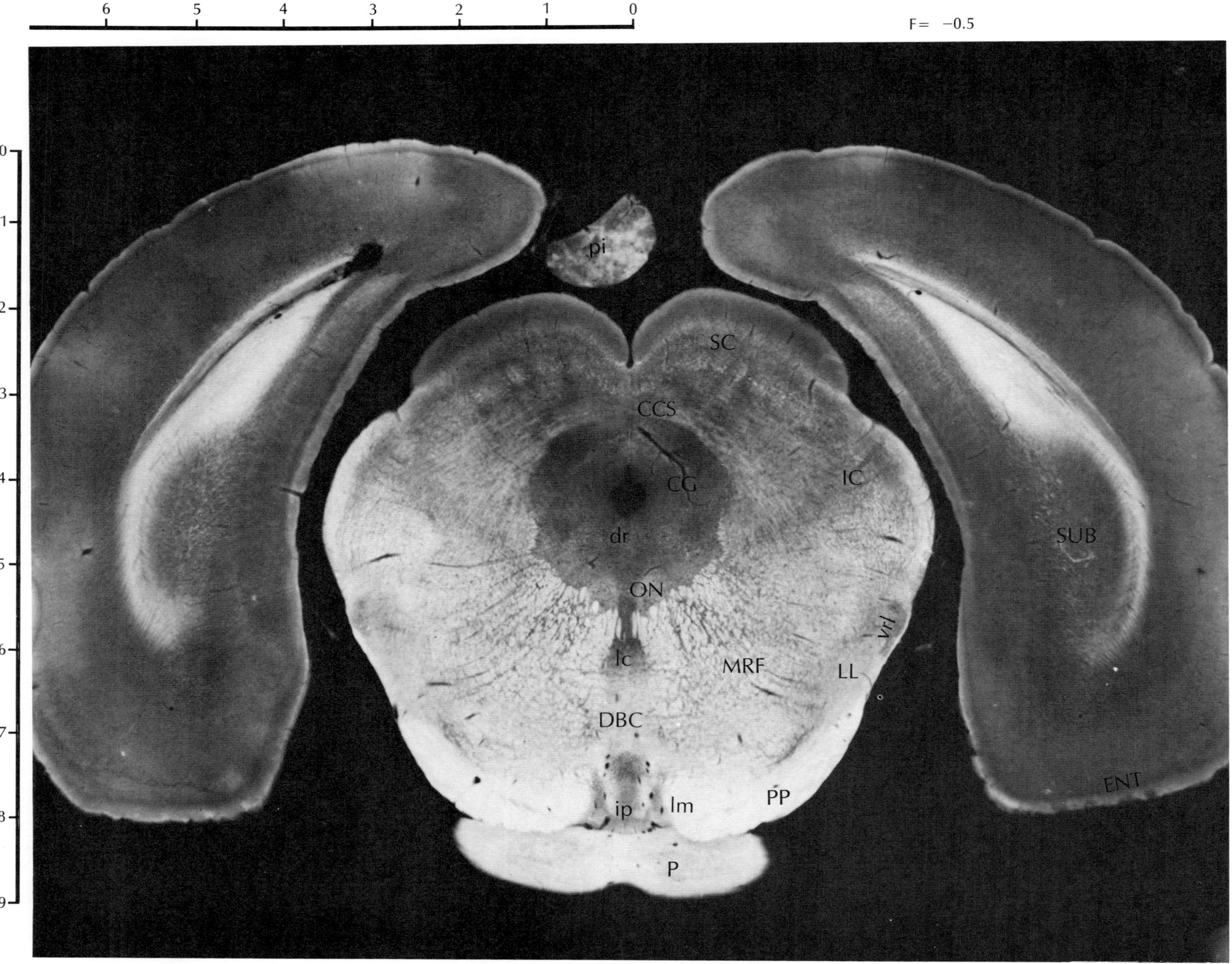

F= −0.5
pi
SC
CCS
CG
IC
dr
ON
VII
SUB
IC
MRF
LL
DBC
ip
lm
PP
P
ENT

Fig. 4-15

INFERIOR COLLICULUS:
hyperkinesia
hyperextension of the head
MEDIAN RAPHE AREA:
visual discrimination deficit
vestibulo-kinesthetic
  discrimination deficit
maze deficit
hyperkinesia
aphagia-adipsia
abnormality of gait
defective labyrinthine reflex
LATERAL LEMNISCAL AREA:
hyperkinesia
aphagia-adipsia
jerky head movements
abnormality of gait
VENTROMEDIAL PONTOMESENCEPHALIC
RETICULAR FORMATION:
visual discrimination deficit
vestibulo-kinesthetic
  discrimination deficit
card displacement deficit
maze deficit
active avoidance deficit
escape response deficit
hyperkinesia
aphagia-adipsia
abnormality of gait
defective labyrinthine reflex
high mortality rate
CG—central gray
DBC—decussation of brachium
  conjunctivum
dr—nucleus dorsalis raphes
IC—inferior colliculus
lm—medial lemniscus
LL—lateral lemniscus
mr—nucleus medianus raphes
MMRF—ponto-mesencephalic
  reticular formation
P—pons
PP—cerebral peduncle
SC—superior colliculus

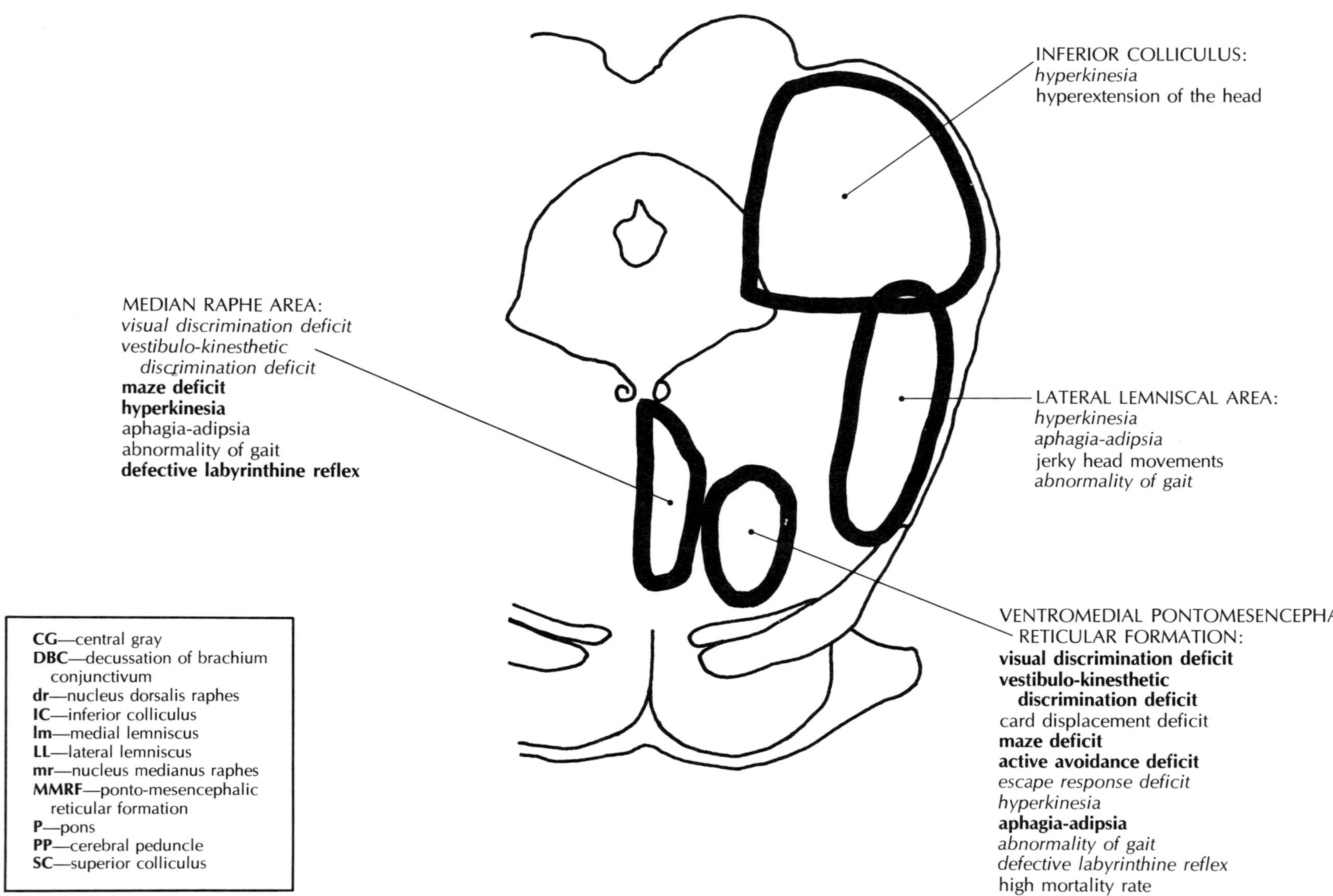

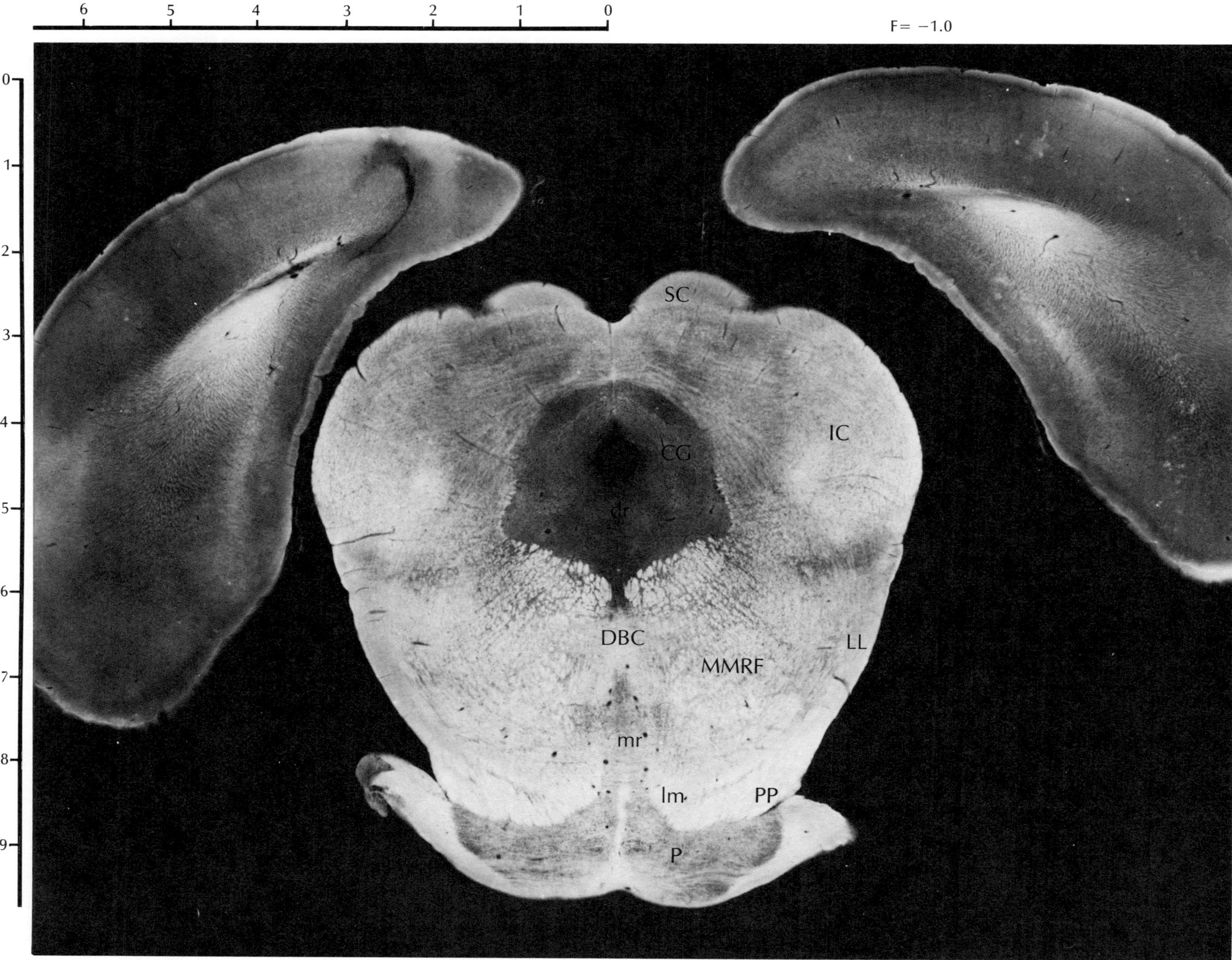

F= −1.0
SC
IC
CG
dr
DBC
LL
MMRF
mr
lm
PP
P

Fig. 4-16

PONTINE RETICULAR FORMATION:
visual discrimination deficit
vestibulo-kinesthetic
  discrimination deficit
card displacement deficit
maze deficit
active avoidance deficit
obstinate progression
hyperkinesia
abnormality of gait
defective labyrinthine reflex

BC—brachium conjunctivum
CG—central gray
IC—inferior colliculus
LL—lateral lemniscus
lm—medial lemniscus
mr—nucleus medianus raphes
ndt—dorsal tegmental nucleus
  of von Gudden
nvt—nucleus ventralis tegmenti
P—pons
PYT—pyramidal tract
rpo—nucleus reticularis
  pontis oralis
tpo—nucleus tegmenti pontis

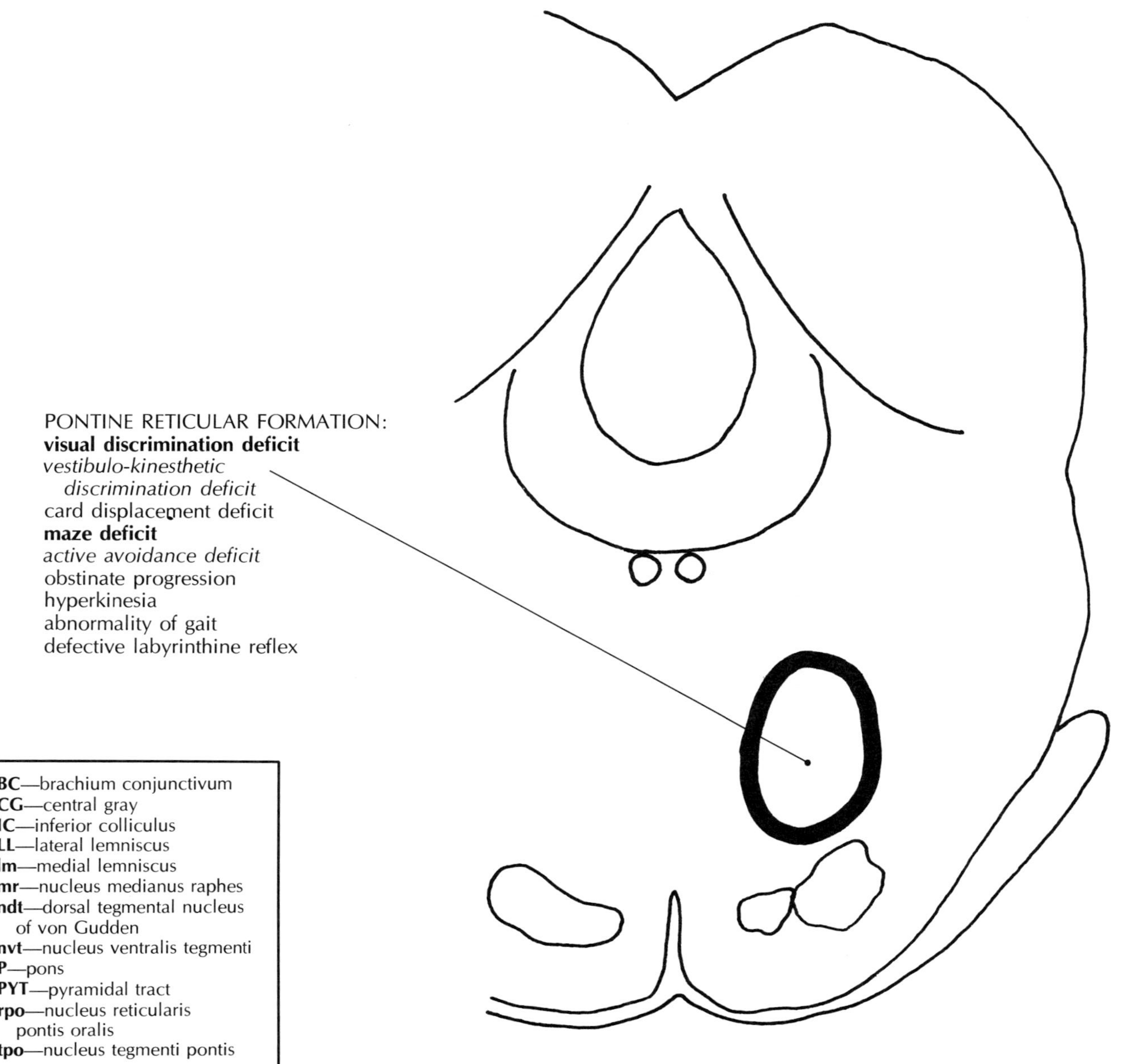

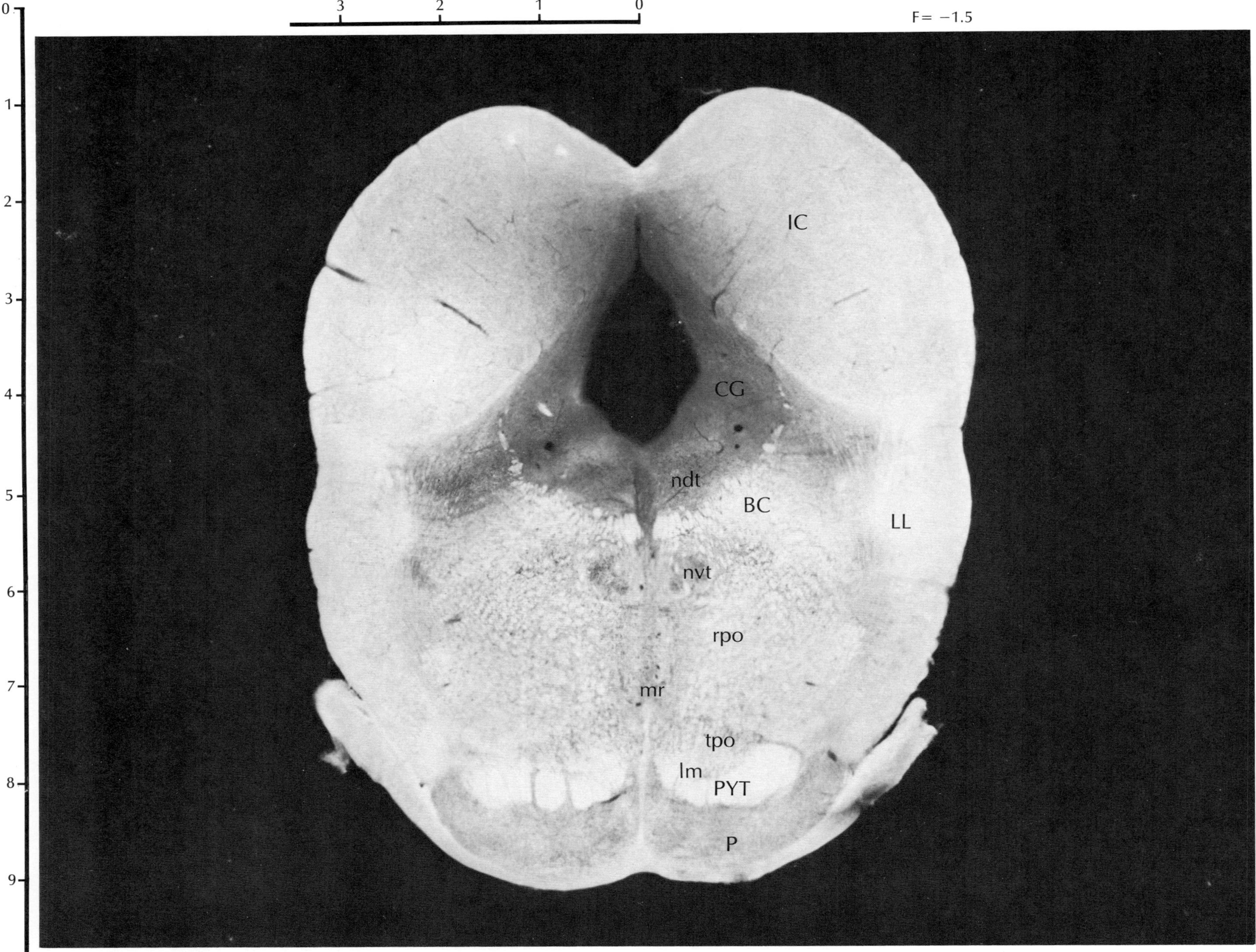

F = −1.5
IC
CG
ndt
BC
LL
nvt
rpo
mr
tpo
lm
PYT
P

5. MAPS OF SPECIFIC DEFICITS

LIST OF DEFICITS AND CORRESPONDING MAPS

MAP KEY

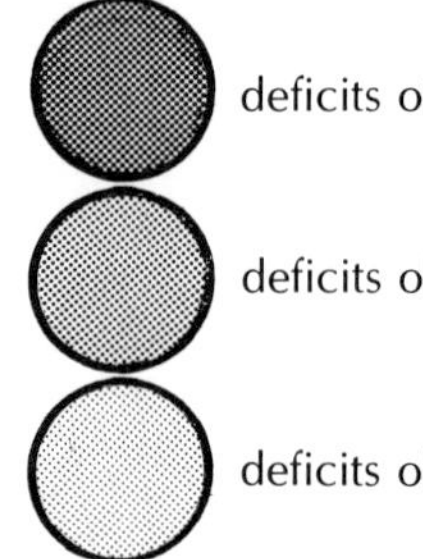

deficits observed in 75–100% of cases

deficits observed in 50–74% of cases

deficits observed in 25–49% of cases

ABBREVIATIONS

AC	anterior cingulate	OLF	olfactory bulb
AMY	amygdala	PAR	parietal cortex
AT	anterior thalamus	PC	posterior cingulate
CB	cerebellum	PF	parafascicular nucleus
CG	central gray	PMRF	pontomesencephalic reticular formation
CMFB	caudal medial forebrain bundle	PR	prerubral area
EPN	entopeduncular nucleus	PRET	pretectal area
ESA	entorhino-subicular area	PRF	pontine reticular formation
FC	frontal cortex	PRRF	postrubal reticular formation
HIP	hippocampus	RCP	rostral caudoputamen
GP	globus pallidus	RMFB	rostral medial forebrain bundle
IC	inferior colliculus	RN	red nucleus
IPCT	interpedunculo-central tegmental area	SC	superior colliculus
LG	lateral geniculate body	SCA	subcollicular area
LLA	lateral lemniscal area	SEP	septal area
LPN	lateral pedunculo-nigral area	SN	substantia nigra
LT	lateral thalamus	SNRF	supranigral reticular formation
MB	mamillary bodies	SOH	medial supraoptic hypothalamus
MCP	middle caudoputamen	SRRF	suprarubral reticular formation
MDRF	mesodiencephalic reticular formation	ST	subthalamus
MDT	dorsomedial thalamus	VLRF	ventrolateral midbrain reticular formation
MR	median raphe nuclei	VMH	ventromedial hypothalamus
NAS	nucleus accumbens septi	VMT	ventromedial thalamus
NP	nucleus posterior	VT	ventral thalamus
OTC	occipito-temporal cortex	VTA	ventral tegmental area

Fig. 5–1
VISUAL DISCRIMINATION DEFICIT

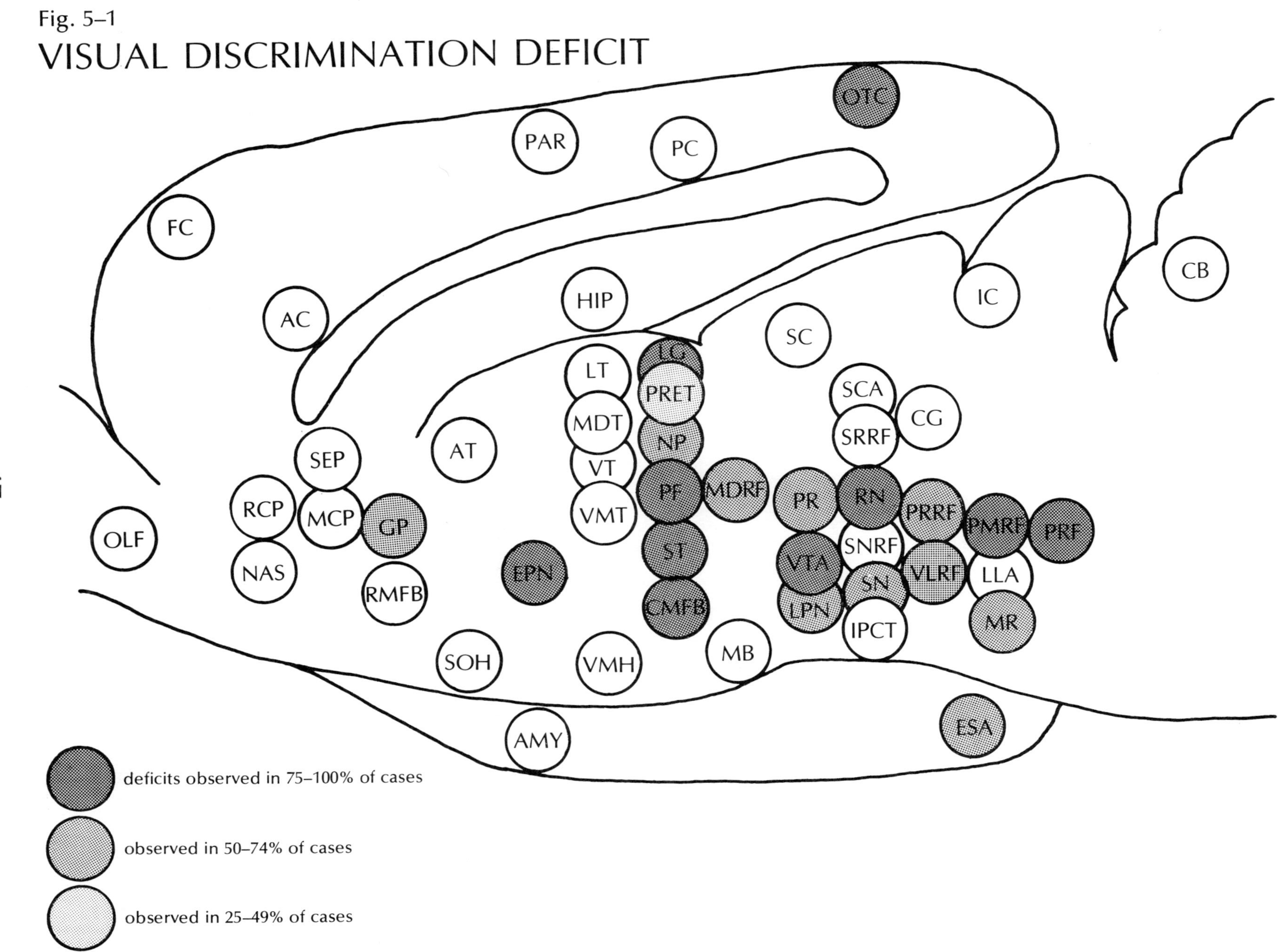

47

Fig. 5–2
VESTIBULO-KINESTHETIC DISCRIMINATION DEFICIT

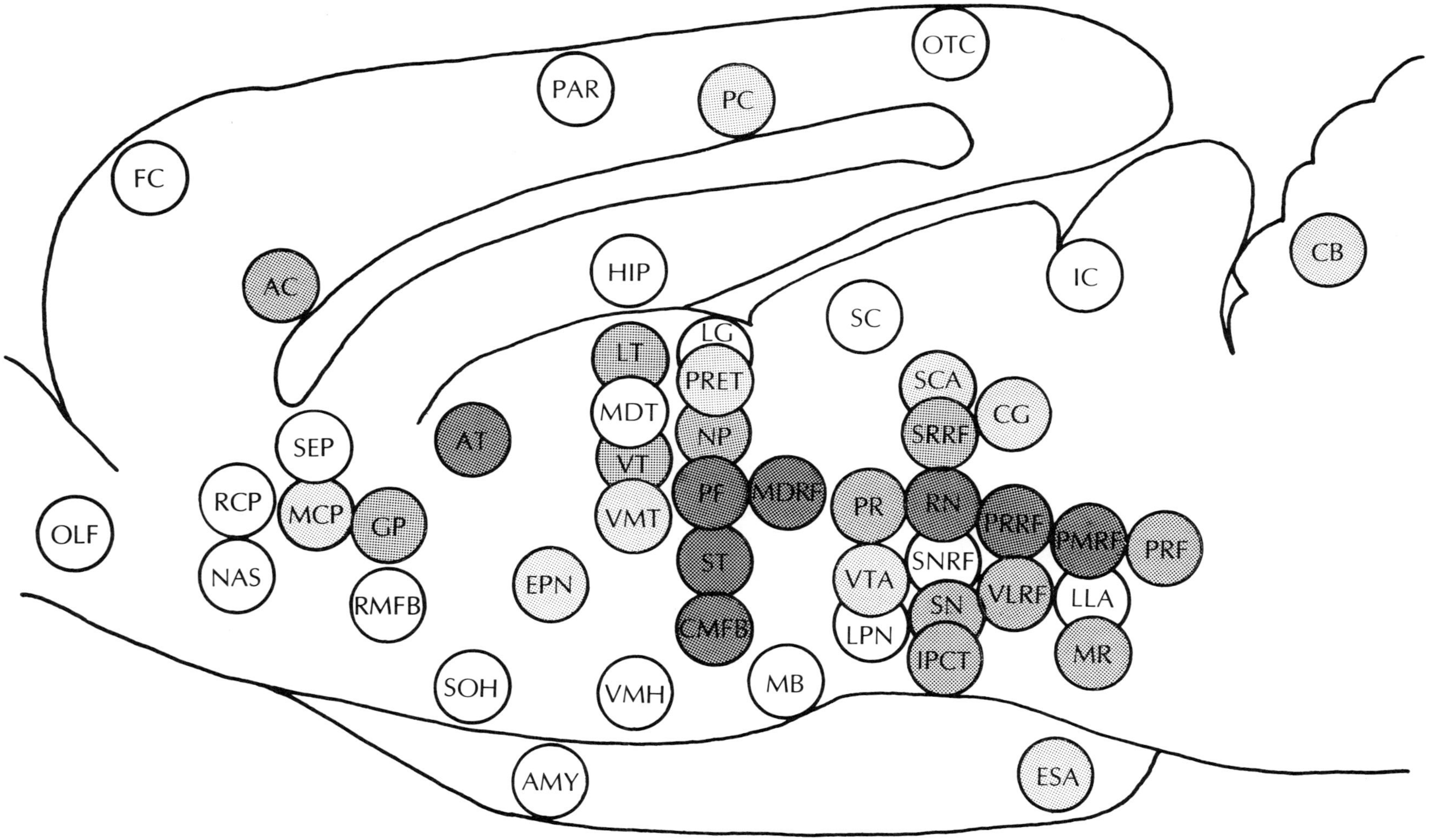

Fig. 5-3
CARD DISPLACEMENT DEFICIT

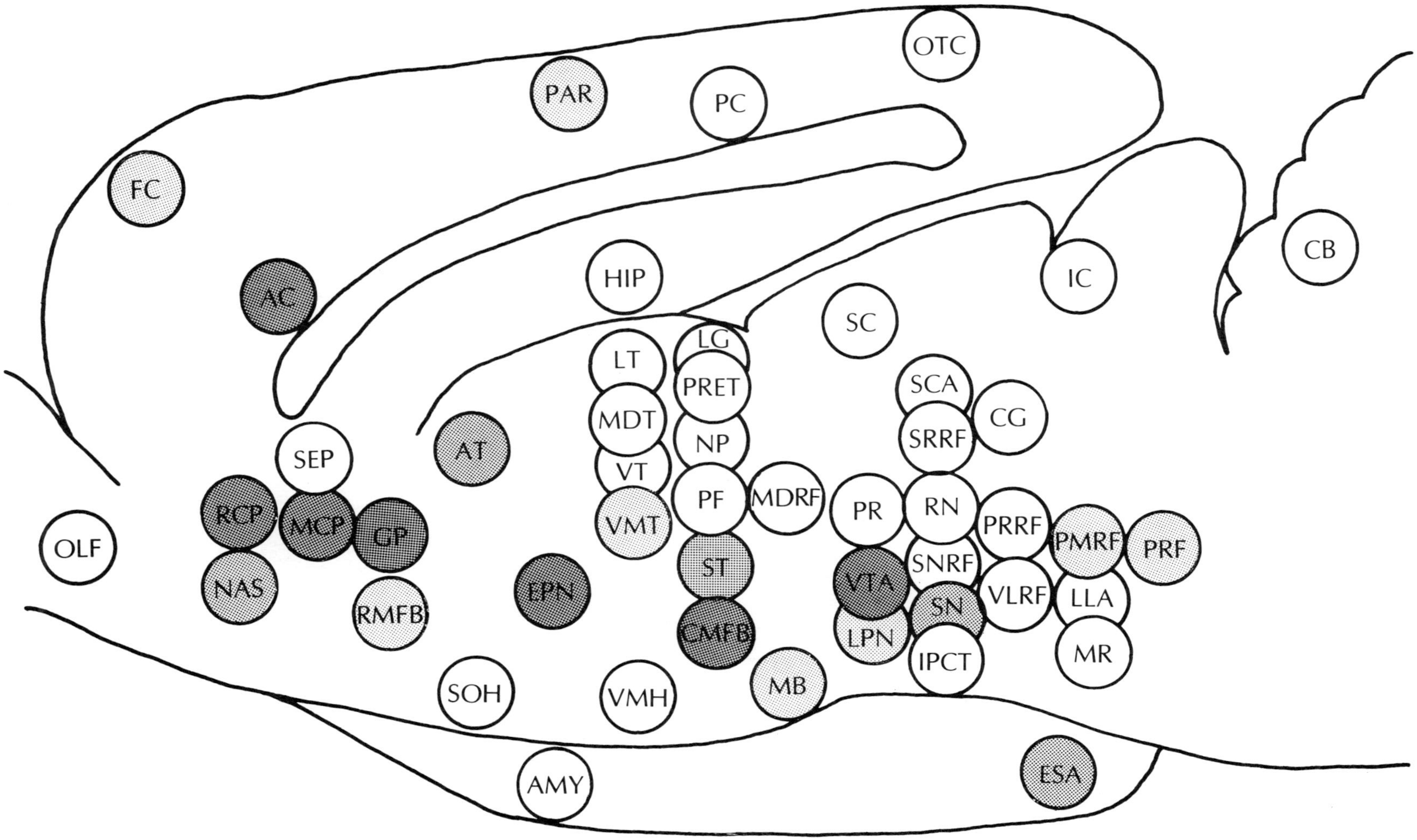

49

Fig. 5-4
MAZE DEFICIT

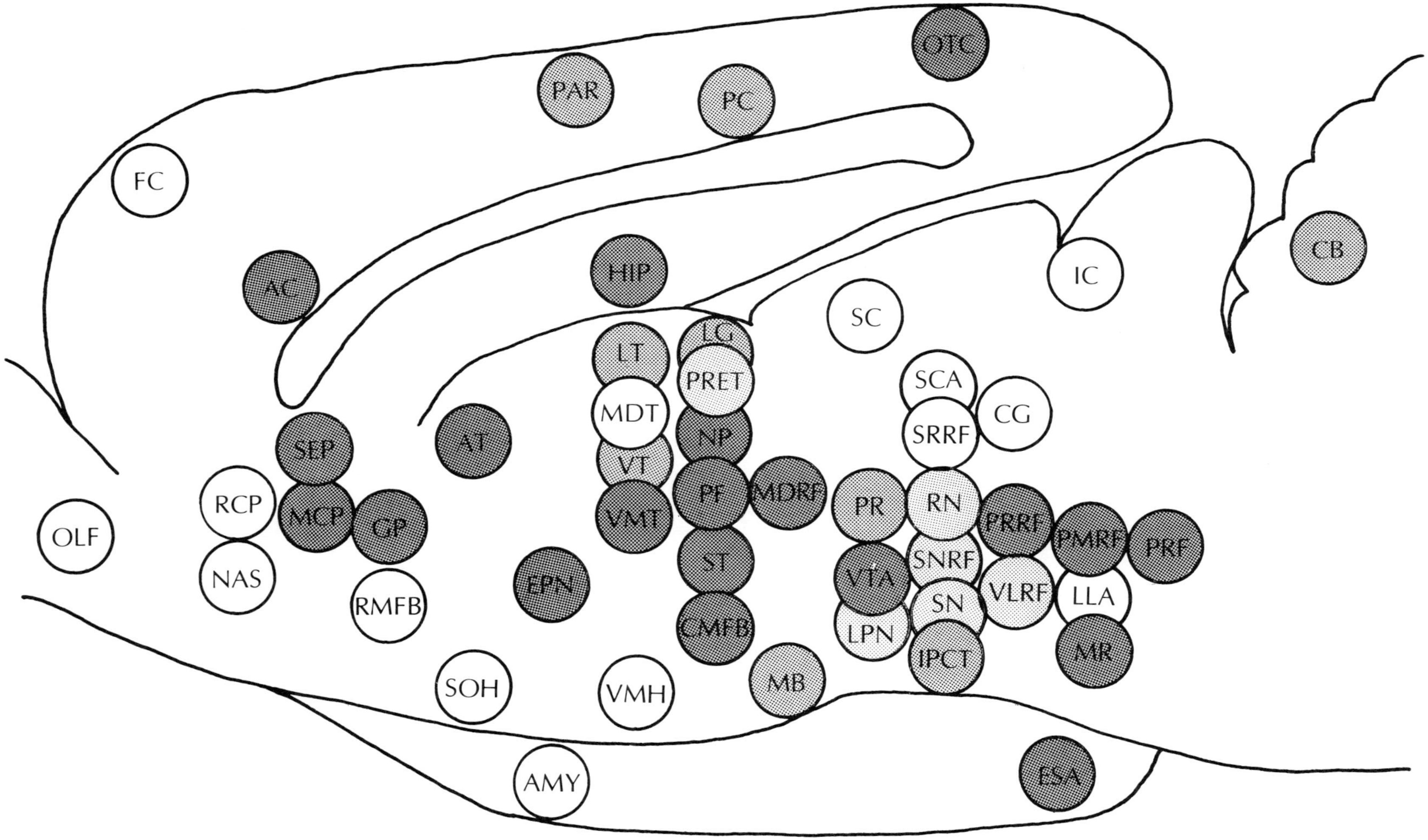

Fig. 5–11
HYPERSENSITIVITY

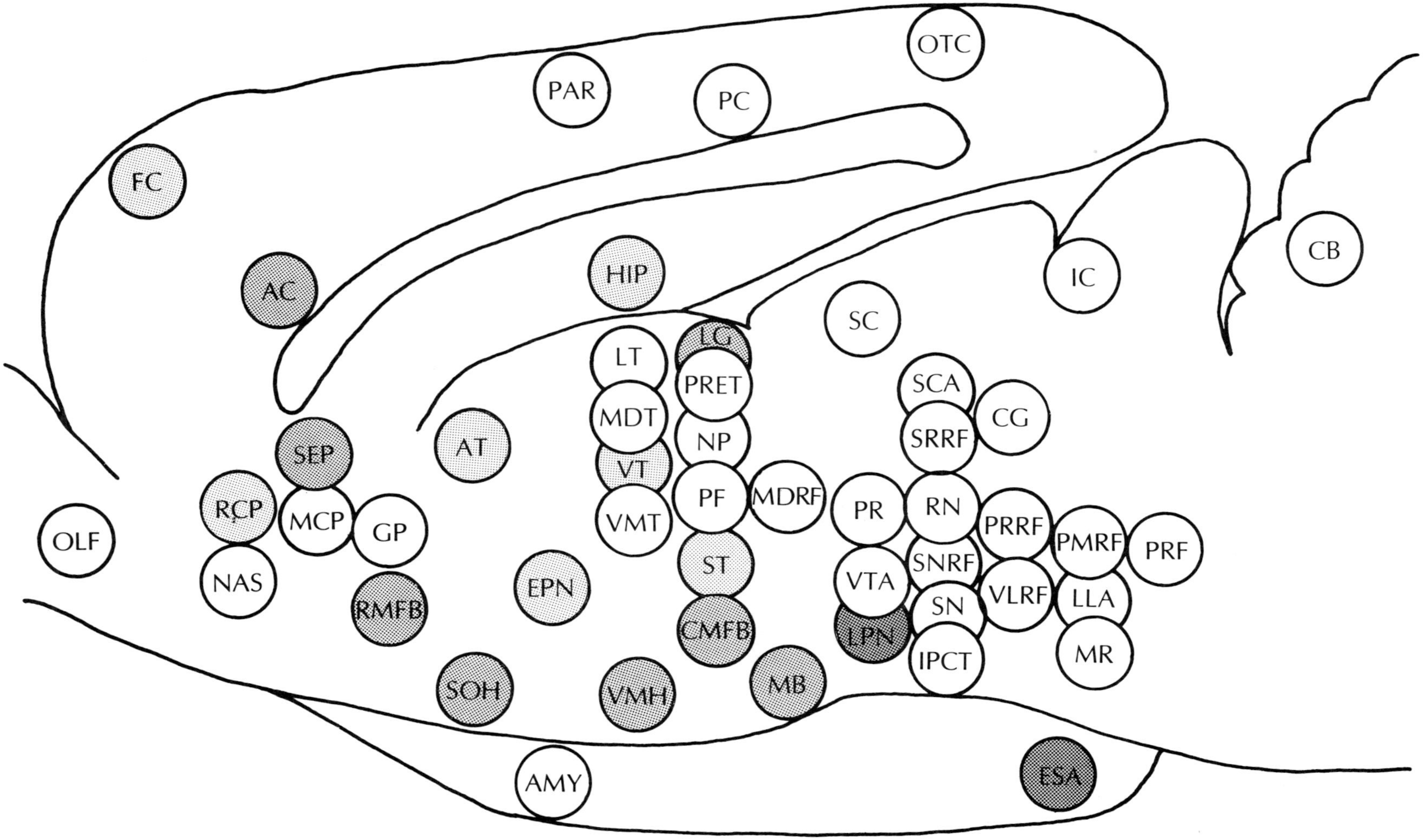

58

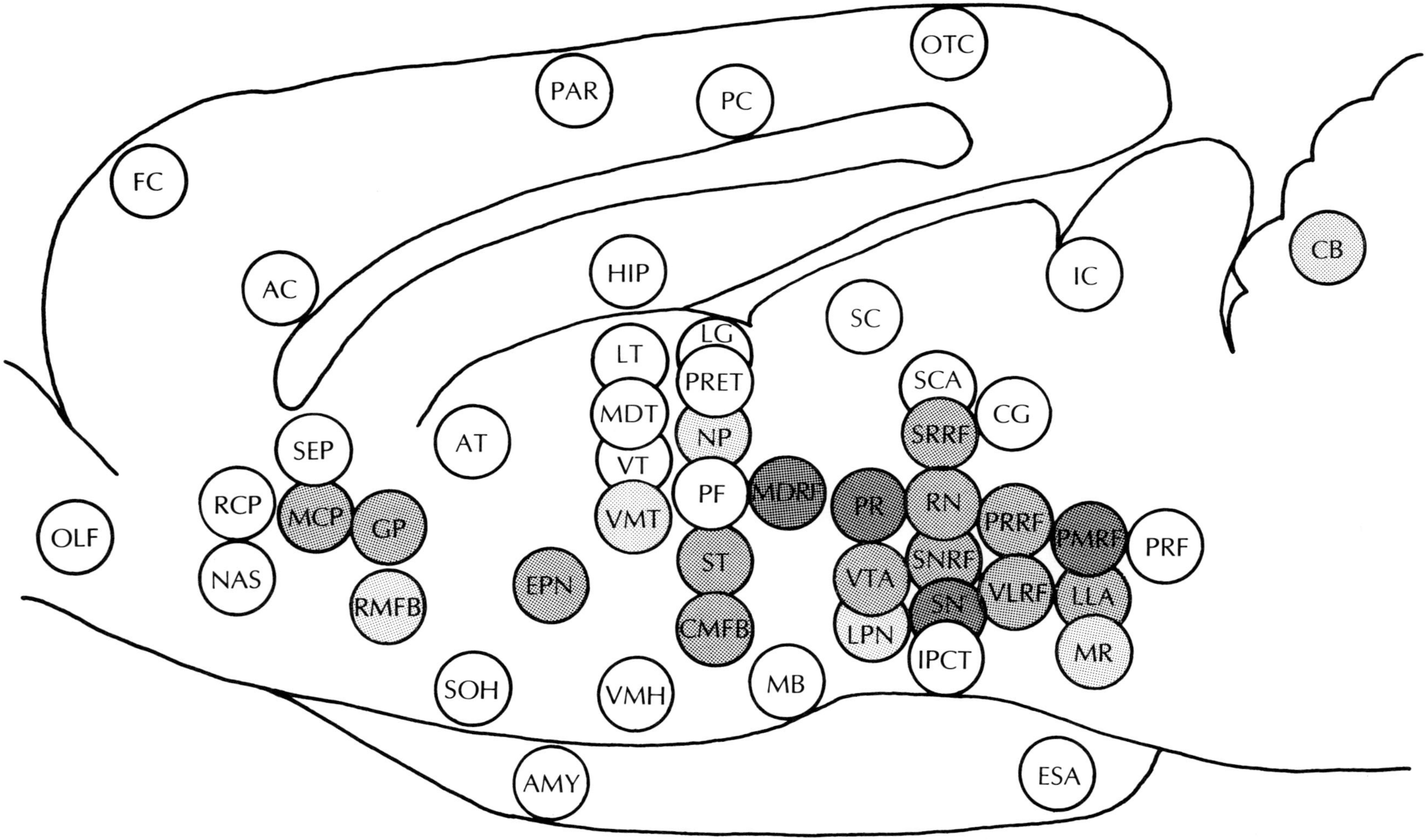

Fig. 5–13
HYPERPHAGIA

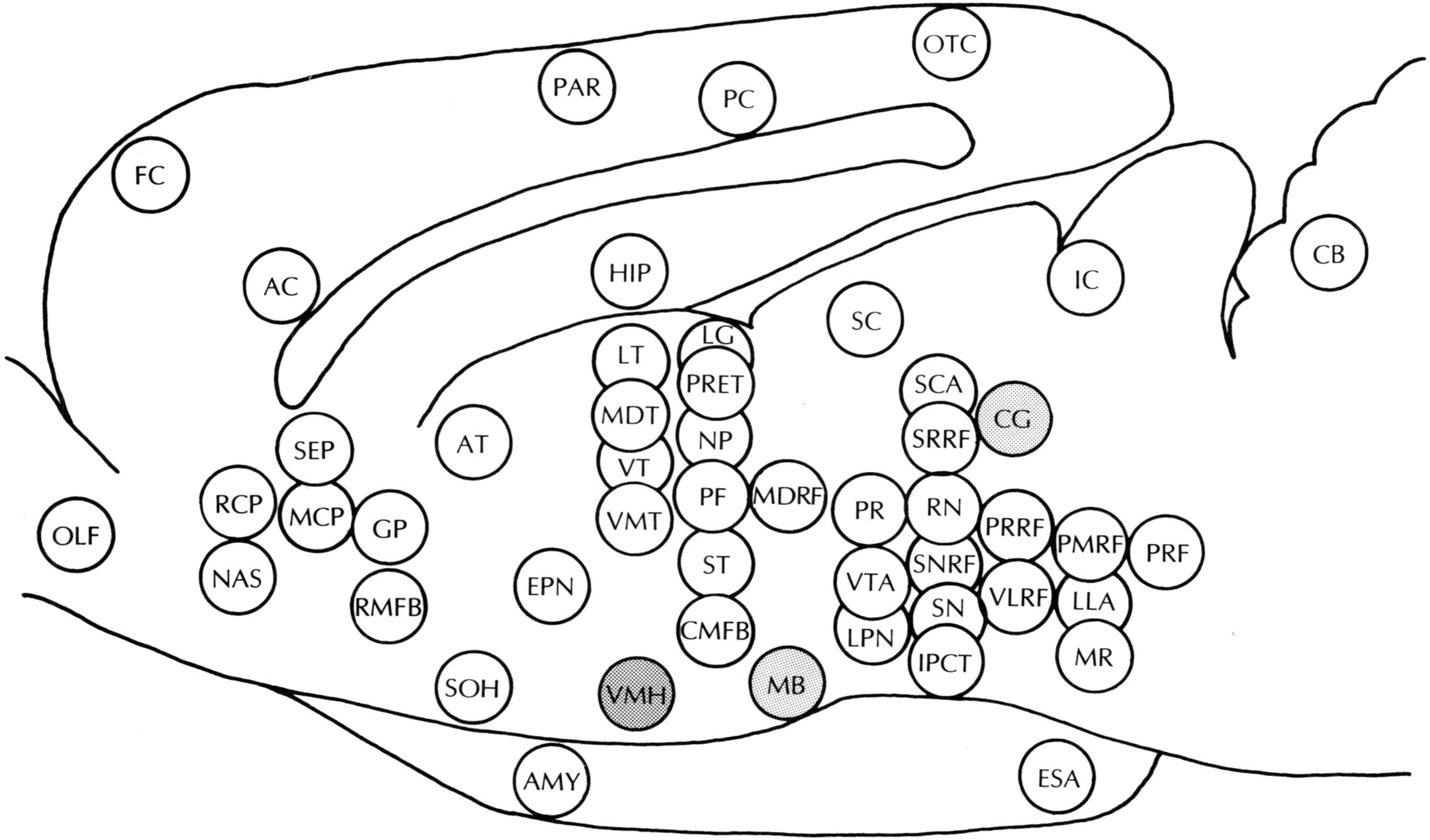

59

Fig. 5-14

AGGRESSIVENESS

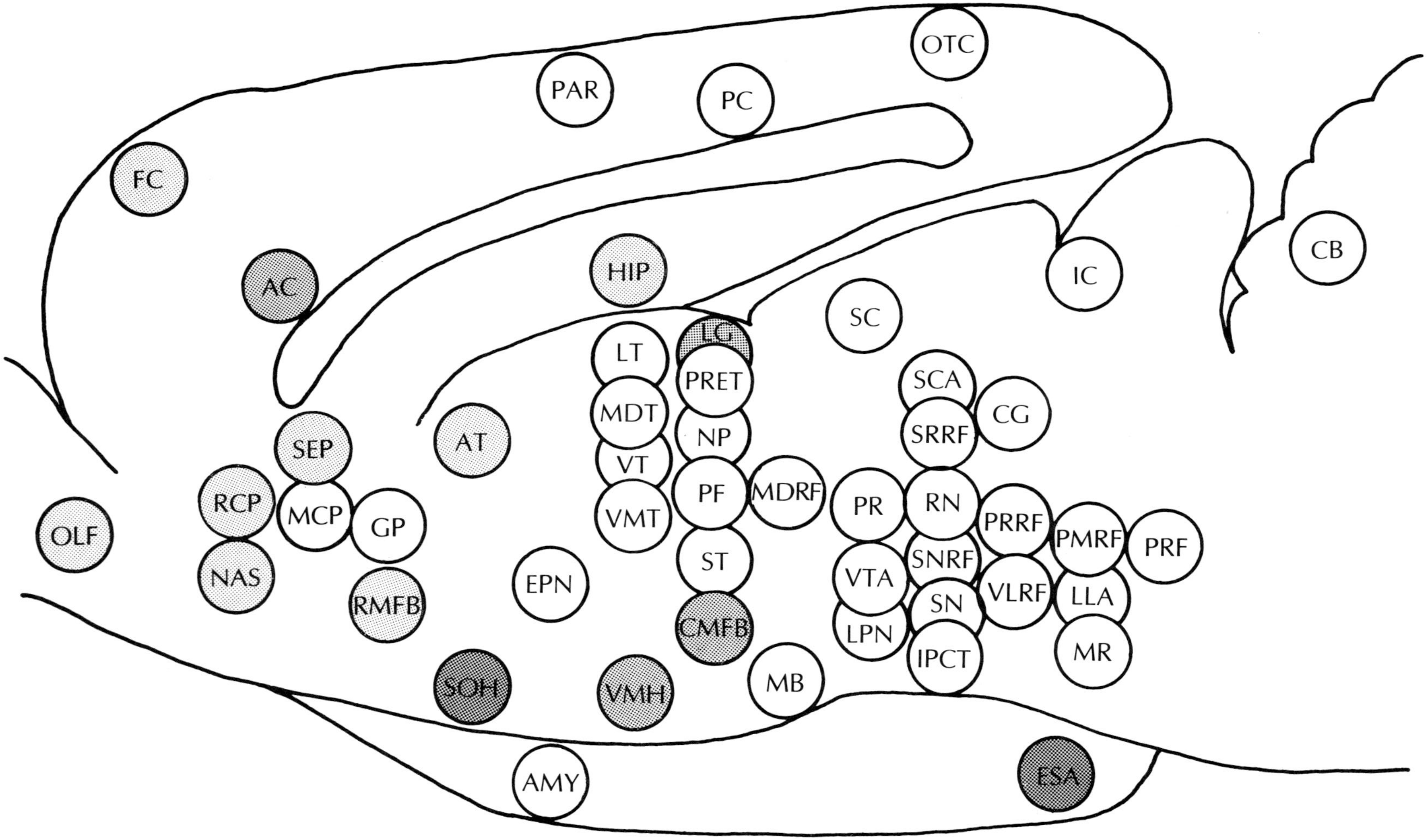

60

Fig. 5-15
JERKY HEAD MOVEMENTS

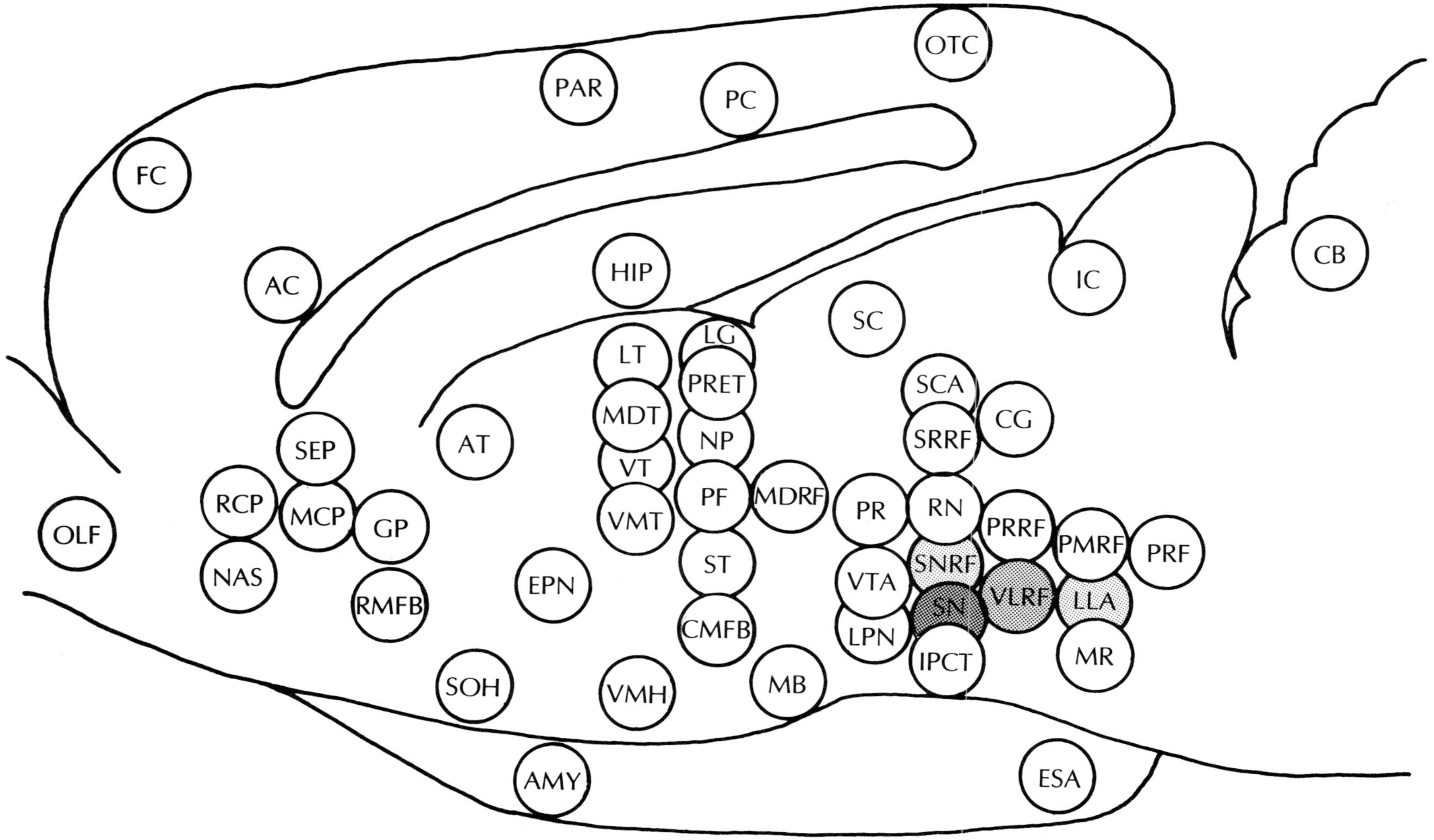

CB
IC
OTC
SC
SCA
CG
SRRF
RN
PRRF
PMRF
PRF
LLA
MR
ESA
VLRF
SNRF
SN
IPCT
PR
VTA
LPN
MDRF
MB
PC
LG
PRET
NP
PF
ST
CMFB
HIP
LT
MDT
VT
VMT
VMH
PAR
AMY
EPN
AT
SOH
GP
RMFB
SEP
MCP
RCP
NAS
AC
FC
OLF

Fig. 5-16

HYPEREXTENSION OF THE HEAD

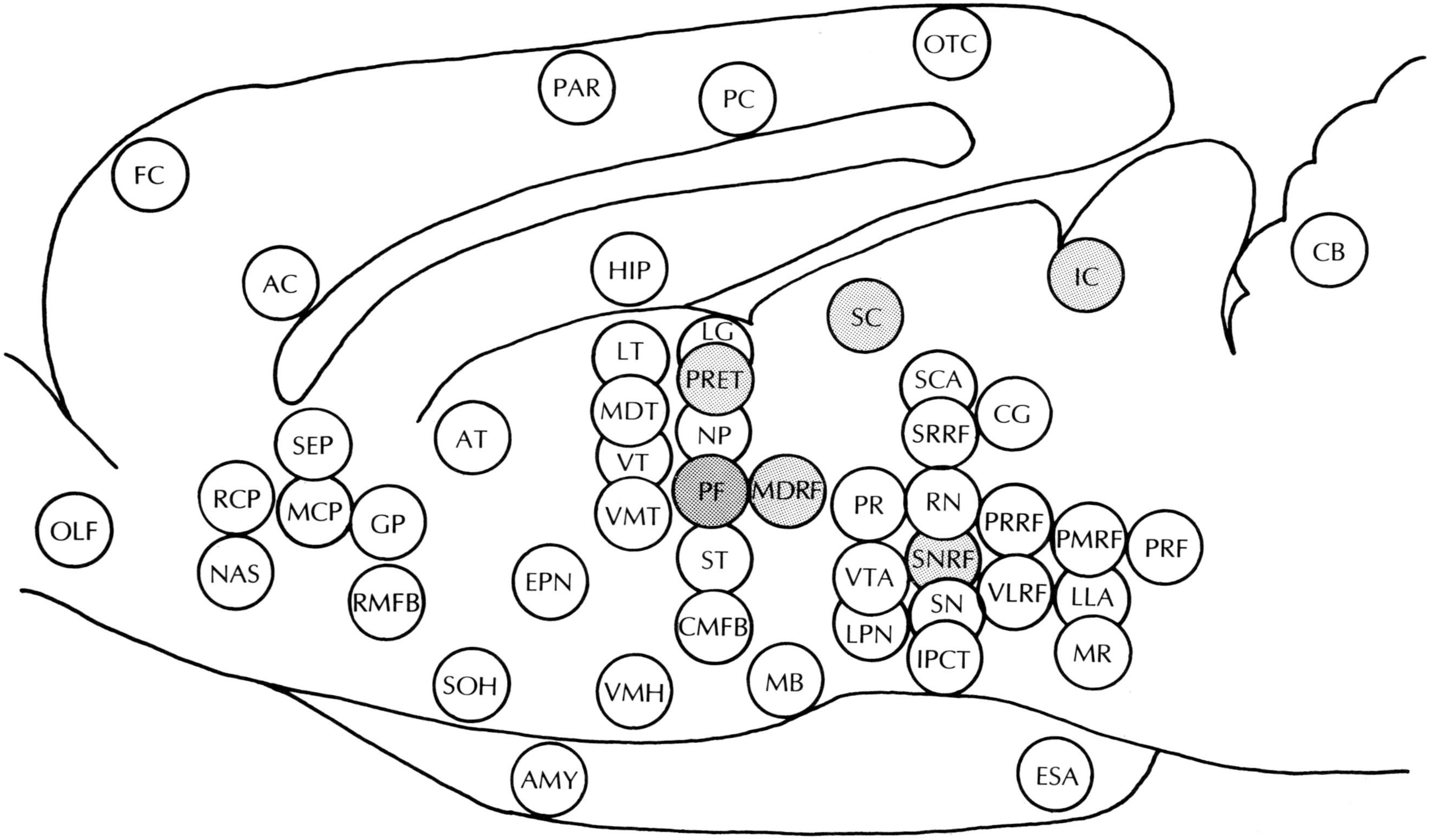

Fig. 5-17
ABNORMALITY OF GAIT

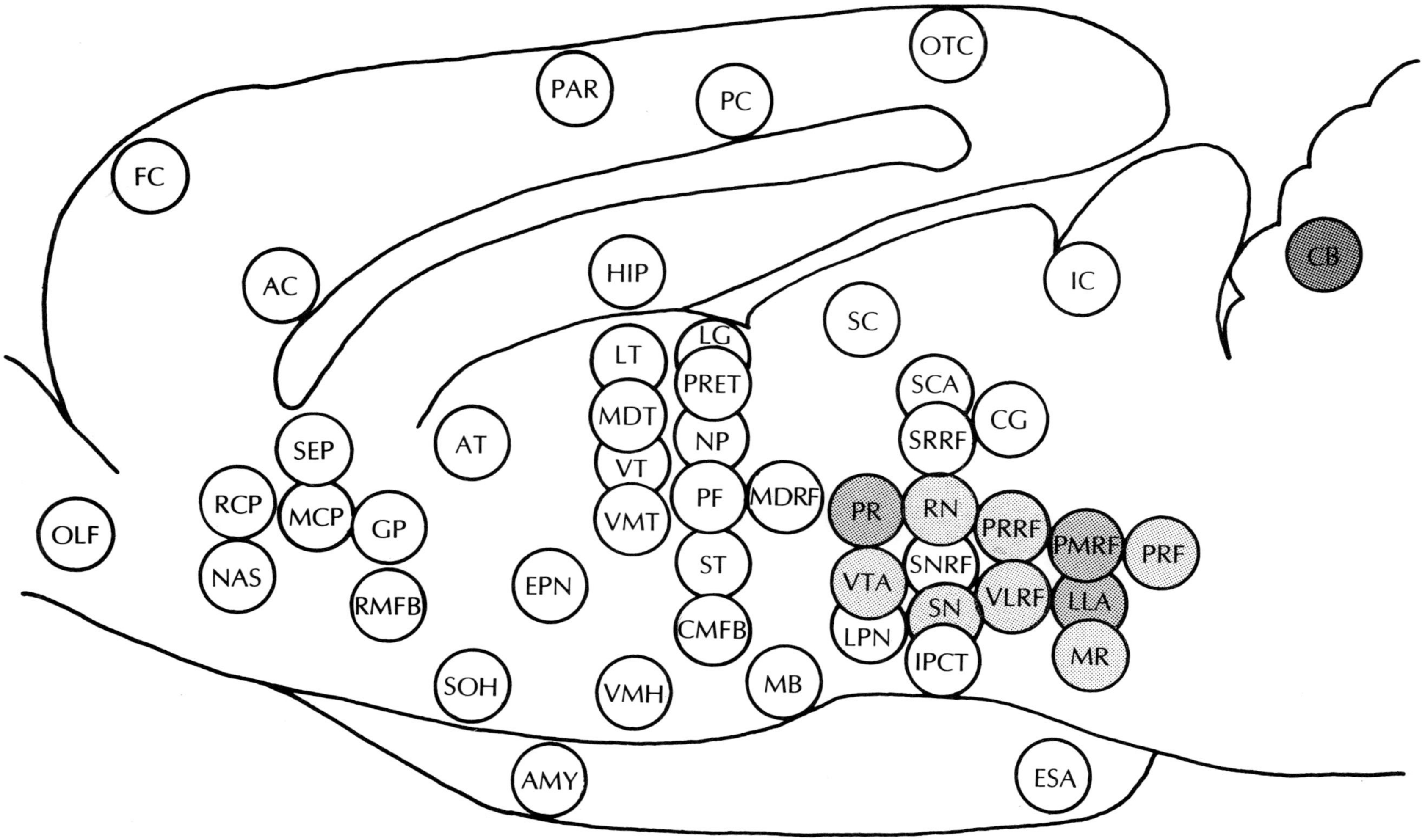

Fig. 5-18 SOMNOLENCE

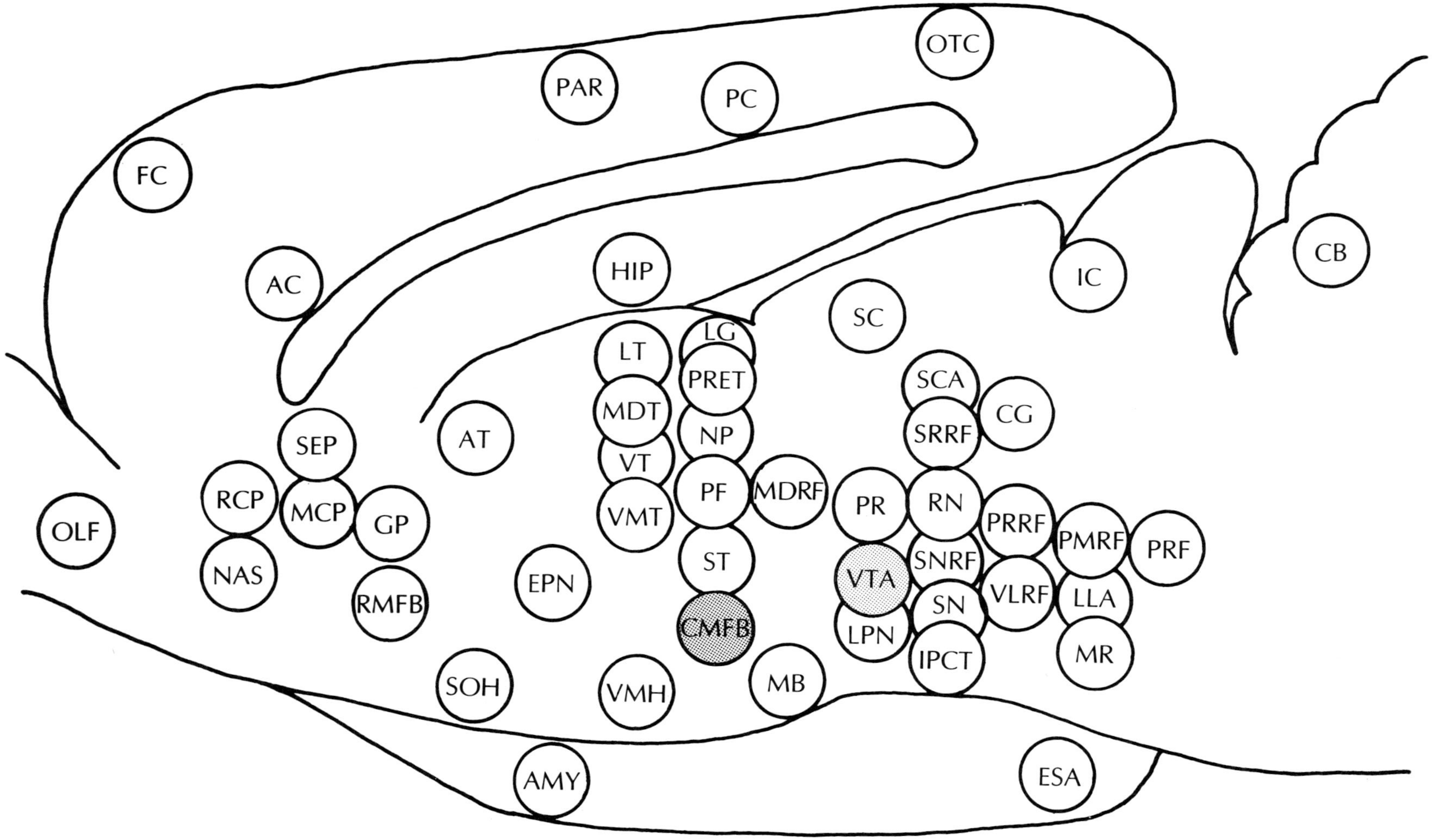

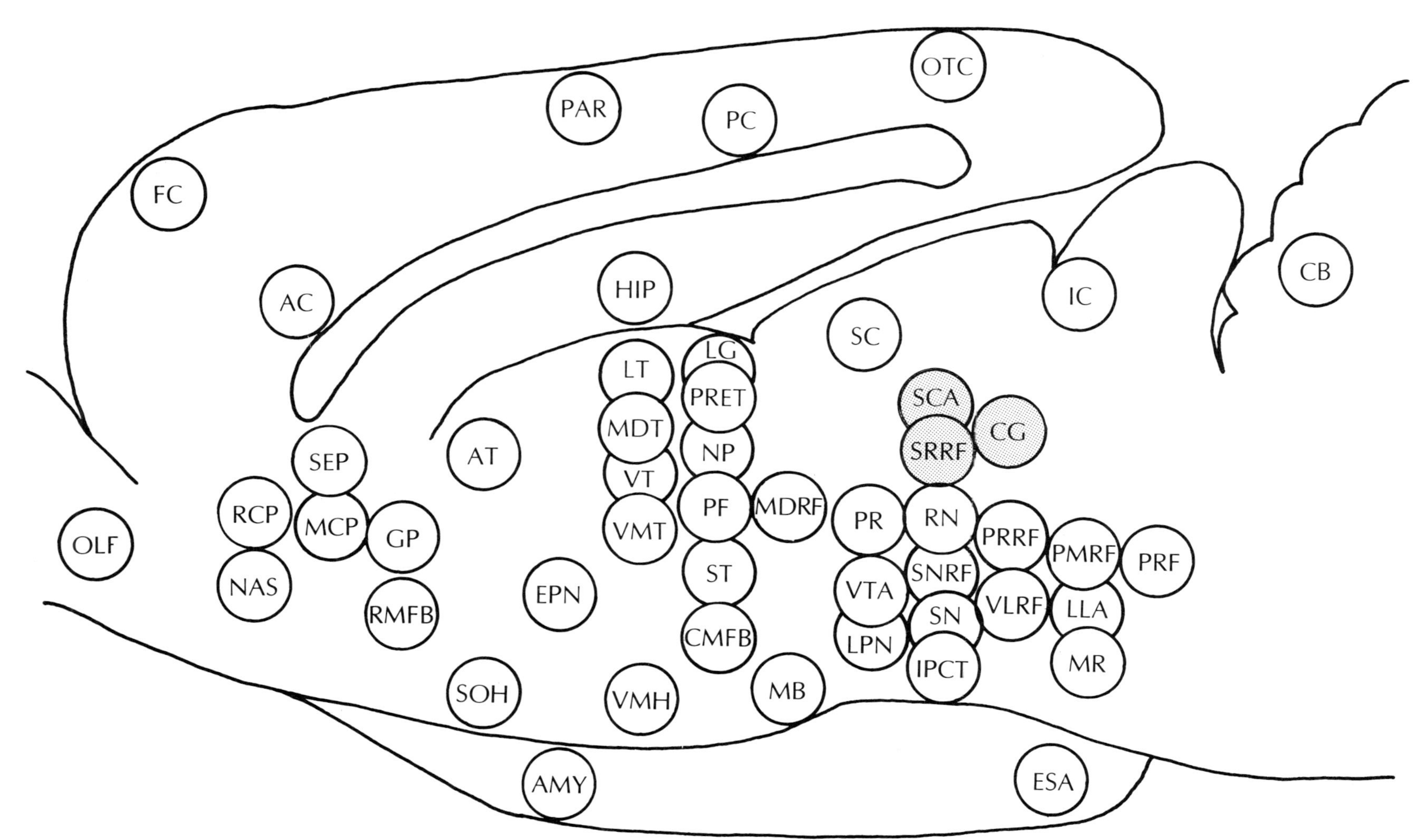

Fig. 5–19
COMA

65

Fig. 5-20

DEFECTIVE PUPILLOCONSTRICTOR REFLEX

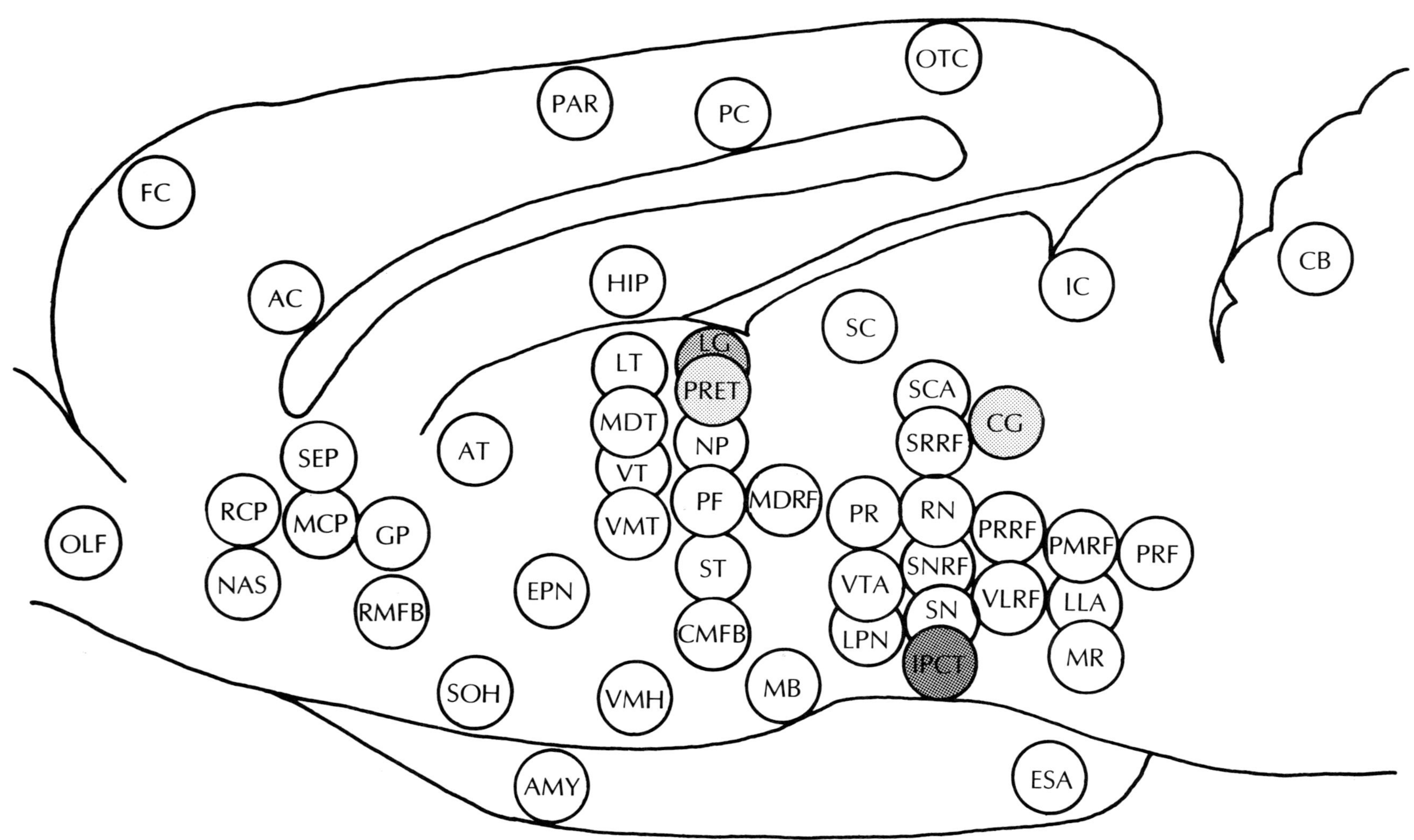

Fig. 5-21 DEFECTIVE LABYRINTHINE REFLEX

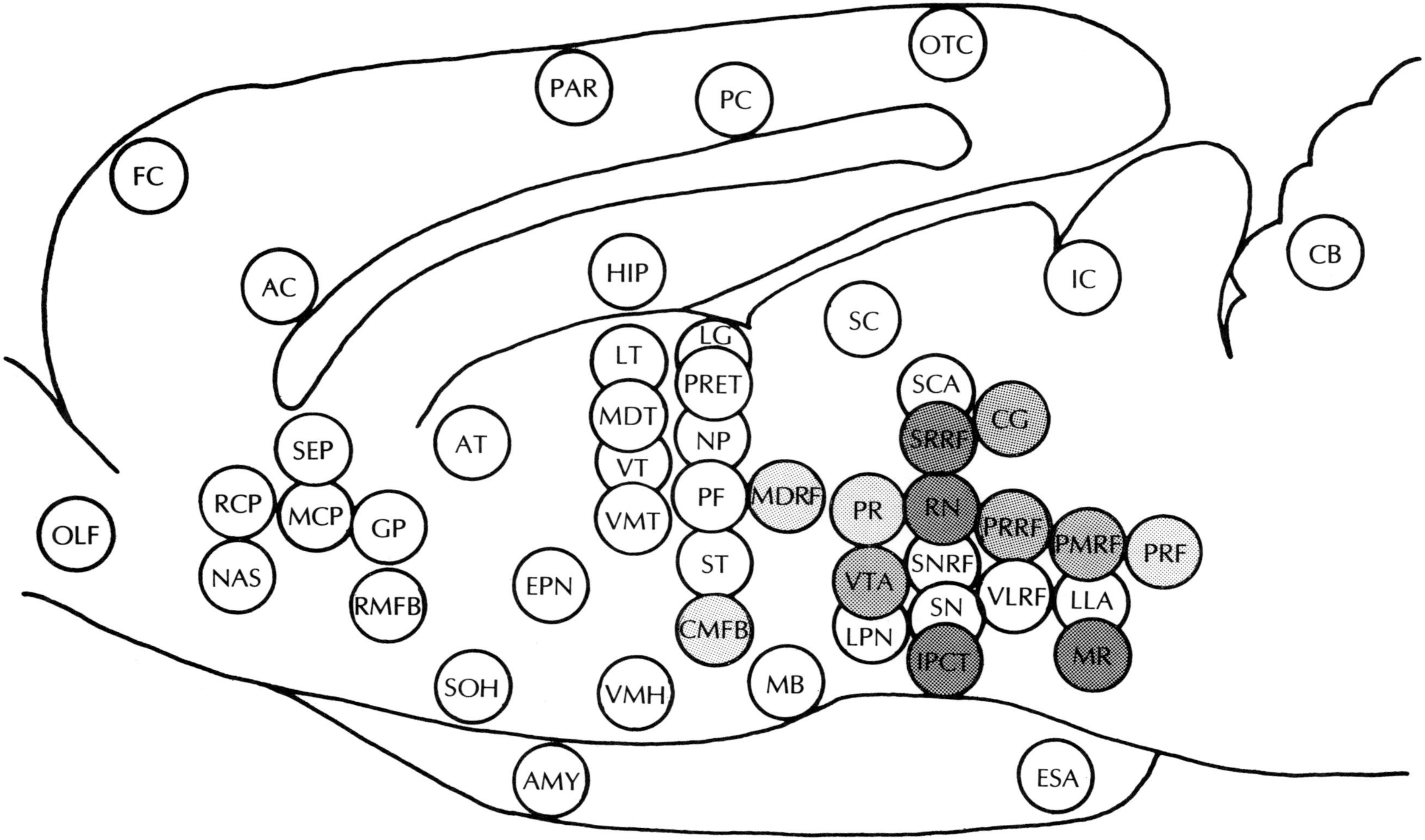

Fig. 5–22
HIGH MORTALITY RATE

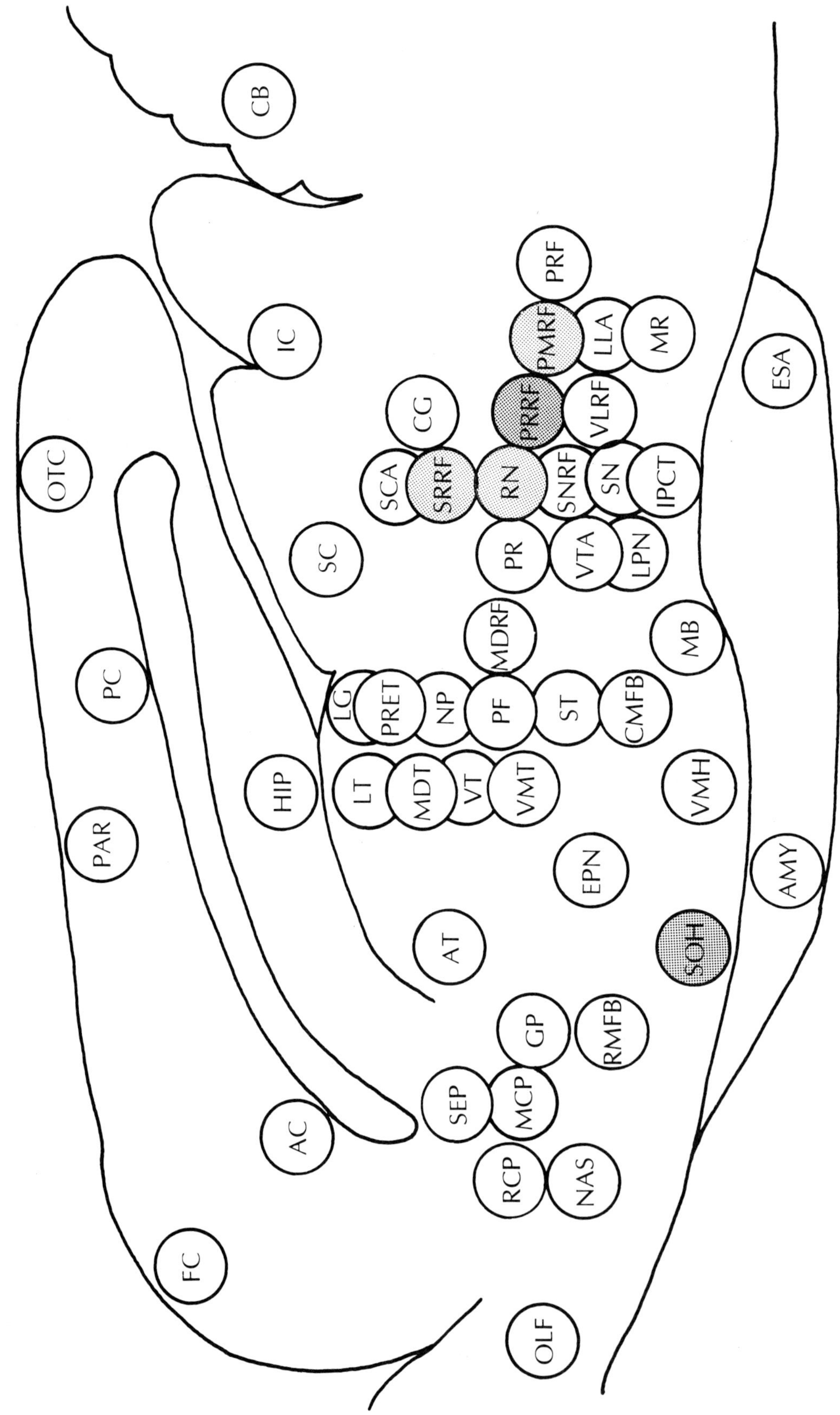

6. INTERPRETING THE BEHAVIORAL ATLAS

HOW TO INTERPRET LESION DATA

As pointed out in Section 1, the primary weakness of the lesion method centers on the fact that any given physiological, behavioral, or mental deficit associated with destruction of a specific brain area is subject to many different interpretations. Some of the difficulties encountered in the interpretation of lesion-induced behavioral losses may be appreciated by examining the syndrome arising from damage to the caudal portion of the medial forebrain bundle in the rat (see Fig. 4-9). Note that the specific deficits range from disturbances in an assortment of previously learned habits to disorders in activity, ingestive behaviors, and responsiveness to tactile stimuli. While these data are a source of clues concerning the functions of the caudal portion of the medial forebrain bundle, they do not provide a solid base from which to draw definitive conclusions. The findings are open to the following questions.

1. Can this complex syndrome be explained on the basis of a single dysfunction or does it reflect a disturbance in a wide variety of elementary functions that are dissociable from one another?
2. Which specific disorders arise from damage to cells intrinsic to this region of the hypothalamus and which arise from damage to pathways coursing through this region?
3. Do some (or all) of these behavioral disorders arise from secondary chemical effects? It is known, for example, that damage to the caudal portion of the medial forebrain bundle causes a reduction in serotonin and noradrenalin levels within the septum, amygdala, hippocampus, and neocortex (Moore & Heller, 1967) and a depletion of dopamine within the caudate nucleus (Ungerstedt, 1971).
4. Would the same syndrome appear if young rats were used rather than adult rats, if a longer recovery period were allowed, or if the lesions were performed in two stages rather than in one stage? (see Stein, Rosen, & Butters, 1974)
5. Are the deficits in learned behaviors due to injury of a pathway or cell group that is utilized in the storage or retrieval of memory traces or are these deficits due to motivational, emotional, or attentional losses?
6. Are the disturbances in ingestive behaviors due to destruction of hunger and thirst "centers" (Stellar, 1954), sectioning of critical sensorimotor pathways (Marshall & Teitelbaum, 1974; Zeigler & Karten, 1974), or interference with a general arousal mechanism (Ungerstedt, 1971)?

Questions of this sort are not peculiar to the investigation of the medial forebrain bundle; they may arise in connection with lesion data obtained on virtually any part of the central nervous system. Unfortunately, answers to most of these questions are not easily acquired, nor will they necessarily guarantee a final determination of the unique functions of a specific brain area (see Webster, 1973). In order to achieve this, converging data from many different sources, including neurophysiological, neurochemical, and neuroanatomical studies, are needed.

How, then, does one interpret data gathered by the lesion method? First of all, it should be emphasized that no helpful hints concerning the specialized functions of a discrete area of the brain can be found in the behavioral consequences of damage to that area *unless other brain areas have been similarly examined.* Conceivably, the same pattern of behavioral deficits might appear with damage to almost any part of the brain. If, however, the deficits following a lesion to structure A can not be duplicated with a lesion to structure B (assuming that the lesions are of equal size), then at least one inference can be made about the possible functions of structure A. This inference is that structure A is more centrally involved than structure B in the expression of the behavior that is disorganized by a lesion to structure A.

Obviously, the significance of such an inference depends upon a number of factors. First, it is more meaningful when structure A and structure B reside at the same gross level of the nervous system—the neocortex (frontal ablation versus parietal ablation), the thalamus (anterior thalamic lesion versus posterior thalamic lesion), the midbrain (red nucleus lesion versus substantia nigra lesion), etc. Second, the inference increases in significance when it is demonstrated that the lesion-induced deficits arise from destruction of nerve cells intrinsic to structure A rather than from interference with extraneous fiber systems passing through structure A. Third, the significance of the inference is strengthened by the degree to which the behavioral deficits are localized to structure A. Finally, the inference takes on added significance to the extent that the behavioral deficits induced by damage to structure A are found to be relatively independent of the age and previous experience of the animal, the type of surgery (one-stage or two-stage operations), the length of the recovery period, and the conditions of observation.

More refined inferences about the involvement of a particular brain structure in the behavior under investigation can conceivably be made by identifying the significant features of the dysfunction. For example, experiments may be carried out to determine if the lesion-induced losses are products of a sensory or motor deficiency, a reduction in arousal, or a disturbance in response inhibition. The difficulty with this approach is that determining the precise character of any lesion-induced dysfunction is a long process that rarely leads to an incontrovertible conclusion. For this reason, further insight is sought in the neurochemical, neuroanatomical, and neurophysiological literature bearing upon the brain structure under investigation. It would be important to know, for example, the behavioral effects of chemical or electrical stimulation of this structure, the nature of the afferent pathways that provide input to the structure, and the behavioral pattern or state of the animal that brings about significant changes in the electrical activity of the structure.

It should be clear at this juncture that localizing a deficit to a specific brain region is far easier than localizing a function to that region. At the same time, it should be recognized that localizing a deficit to a specific brain region is an initial step toward identifying the neural substrates of behavior. The fact that progress toward this goal is impeded by problems of interpretation must be viewed from the perspective that the behavior of living organisms is a highly complex phenomenon and that most fields represented within the behavioral sciences tend to progress at a slow rate because of uncertainties involved in the interpretation of the data (see Pereboom, 1971).

LESION DATA IN SECTION 4
In light of the foregoing considerations, only limited inferences can be made about the syndromes charted in Section 4. Some of the more intriguing inferences of a general nature, along with a few comments and suggestions concerning the interpretation of the data, will be offered.

1. It is instructive to note at the outset that lesion-induced deficits are not all of the same character. From a physiological point of view, it is useful to differentiate between a lesion-induced "release" deficit and a lesion-induced "deficiency" deficit (Kornhuber, 1974). In general, the former refers to some increase in a behavioral or physiological response due to removal or blockage of inhibitory influences. Among the release deficits observed in the current study were hypermetamorphosis, hyperkinesia, hypersensitivity, hyperphagia, aggressiveness, and jerky head movements. A lesion-induced deficiency deficit refers to a decrease in a behavioral or in a physiological response due to removal or blockage of facilitatory influences. Among the deficiency deficits observed in the current study were hypokinesia, aphagia-adipsia, somnolence, and a defective pupilloconstrictor reflex. As might be expected, release and deficiency deficits may profoundly influence the performance of other classes of behavior, such as learned responses.

2. A unique syndrome was correlated with each of the 50 brain areas where lesions were placed (see Section 4). At first glance, this correlation suggests that no two brain areas are identical in their overall involvement in the behavioral and physiological responses investigated in this study. However, it must be noted that electrolytic and aspirative lesions destroy fiber pathways as well as nerve cells and that destruction of the former may account, at least in part, for the uniqueness of the syndromes.

3. Inspection of the various syndromes suggests that the involvement of each brain area in behavioral and physiological processes may be more complex and diffuse than currently conceptualized. Recent textbooks in physiological psychology, for example, typically discuss the lateral geniculate nuclei, pretectal area, and occipital cortex only in relation to the visual system; the brainstem reticular formation only in relation to attention, arousal, and wakefulness; and the caudoputamen, globus pallidus, subthalamus, substantia nigra, and red nucleus only in relation to postural mechanisms. Yet the syndromes arising from lesions to these areas of the brain extended to classes of behavior seemingly unrelated to vision, attention, and posture. Making sense out of the diffuse complexity of most of the syndromes described in Section 4 must await the discovery of the pluralistic circuits by which specialized parts of the brain interact to produce the full spectrum of behavioral patterns that the rat is capable of.

4. Assuming that the number of deficits arising from a lesion to a given brain site is an index of the "functional complexity" of that site, then the results of this behavioral atlas have opened the way to a provisional examination of regional differences in functional complexity. Obviously, conclusions based on any significant regional differences must be made with caution, especially when it is considered that the relative number of deficits listed under a syndrome will probably be a function of such variables as the composition of the test battery, the length of the recovery period, the size of the lesions, and the number of extraneous fiber systems interrupted by the lesions.

In Table 6-1 the 50 different brain sites examined in this study are grouped under one of 10 arbitrary divisions of the brain. The mean number of deficits is shown for each division, together with the brain sites in each division associated with the highest and lowest number of deficits. It can be seen that the brainstem reticular formation and the basal ganglia exhibited the highest degree of functional complexity, while the cortex and the dorsal midbrain exhibited the lowest degree of functional complexity: with the use of the Mann-Whitney test (1947), these division differences in the number of deficits were significant at least at the .05 level. No other division differences were significant, except that between the brainstem reticular formation and the limbic forebrain areas.

The finding that certain brainstem regions exhibit greater functional complexity than cortical or limbic forebrain regions is remarkably consistent with the notions recently advanced by Berntson and Micco (1976). Based on a review of the literature dealing with both the behavioral patterns elicited by brainstem stimulation and the behavioral capacities of decerebrated animals, Berntson and Micco have argued that the brainstem contains those networks of neurons that are fundamental to the expression of many complex and coordinated behavioral patterns characteristic of the species under investigation. Limbic forebrain and neocortical systems are conceived to exert modulating influences on the brainstem and to contribute refinement to the final integration of behavior. According to this conceptualization, brainstem lesions would be expected to

Table 6-1. Regional differences in the total number of deficits (functional complexity)

Brain division[1]	Number of brain sites	Mean	Highest	Lowest
Brainstem reticular formation (MDRF, PR, SNRF, SRRF, VLRF, PRRF, PMRF, and PRF)	8	8.7[2]	PMRF (11)	SRRF and SNRF (7)
Basal ganglia (RCP, NAS, MCP, GP, EPN, ST, VTA, SN, LPN, and RN)	10	8.6[3]	VTA (12)	NAS (4)
Midline midbrain areas (IPCT and MR)	2	6.5	MR (7)	IPCT (6)
Hypothalamus (RMFB, SOH, VMH, CMFB, and MB)	5	6.5	CMFB (13)	SOH (3)
Thalamus (AT, LT, MDT, VT, VMT, LG, PRET, NP, and PF)	9	6.0	AT, VMT, NP, and PRET (8)	LT and DMT (2)
Cerebellum	1	6		
Limbic forebrain areas (OLF, SEP, HIP, ESA, and AMY)	5	5.4	ESA (10)	OLF (3)
Far lateral midbrain area	1	4.0		
Dorsal midbrain area (SC, SCA, CG, and IC)	4	4.0	CG (7)	IC (2)
Cortex (FC, AC, PAR, PC, and OTC)	5	3.8	AC (7)	PC (2)

1. Abbreviations for individual brain sites are the same as those used in Section 5.
2. Differed from the cortex, dorsal midbrain, and limbic forebrain at least at the .05 level.
3. Differed from the cortex and dorsal midbrain at least at the .05 level.

abolish or at least disorganize a greater number of behavioral patterns than would cortical or limbic forebrain lesions. The latter, however, would be expected to produce deficits mainly in the elaboration and control of adaptive response sequences under changing environmental conditions.

5. By focusing on the number of deficits in learned tasks listed under each syndrome, it is possible to examine regional differences in what might be termed "cognitive complexity." Again, one must be cautious in the interpretation of any significant regional differences in cognitive complexity for the reasons mentioned above.

Table 6-2 presents the mean number of deficits in learned tasks for each of the 10 divisions of the brain together with the individual brain sites in each division associated with the highest and lowest number of deficits in learned tasks. As in the case of functional complexity, the basal ganglia and the brainstem reticular formation exhibited the highest degree of cognitive complexity, while the cortex and the dorsal midbrain were among the four divisions exhibiting the lowest degree of cognitive complexity.

This difference in cognitive complexity between the cortex and certain brainstem regions may be taken as evidence favoring the existence of a subcortically induced memory trace (Gastaut, 1958; Penfield & Mathieson, 1974; Thompson, 1965), but other interpretations are certainly possible. For example, it might be argued that certain brainstem lesions abolish "energizing" influences on other cerebral areas (Luria, 1970), thus causing generalized disturbances in retrieval and utilization of stored information. Or, in line with the notions of Berntson and Micco (1976), it might be argued that the disorganization of those species-characteristic behavioral patterns involved in the expression of learned responses lies at the basis of the retention deficits induced by certain brainstem lesions.

6. Discrepancies between the syndromes described in the clinical and experimental literature are not uncommon (see, for example, Isaacson, 1972, and Ploog, 1975) or unexpected, especially when some of the striking anatomical differences between the brains of humans and those of animals are considered (Sarnat & Netsky, 1974). This is not to say that similarities are nonexistent. When we compare the syndromes

Table 6–2. Regional differences in the number of deficits in learned tasks (cognitive complexity)

Brain division	Number of brain sites	Mean	Highest	Lowest
Basal Ganglia	10	4.8[1]	VTA, SN, ST, EPN, and GP (6)	NAS (2)
Brainstem reticular formation	8	4.4[1]	PMRF (6)	SRRF (2)
Cerebellum	1	4		
Thalamus	9	3.7	AT, VMT, NP, PRET, and PF (5)	MDT (1)
Midline midbrain areas	2	3.5	IPCT (4)	MR (3)
Limbic forebrain areas	5	2.8	ESA (6)	OLF (1)
Cortex	5	2.6	AC (4)	FC (1)
Hypothalamus	5	2.4	CMFB (6)	SOH and VMH (0)
Dorsal midbrain area	4	1.5	CG (3)	IC (0)
Far lateral midbrain area	1	0		

1. Differed from the dorsal midbrain and cortex at least at the .05 level.

described in this behavioral atlas with those reported in the clinical literature, some similarities do appear. Table 6-3 presents some of those similarities. It should be noted that correspondence is found at both neocortical and brainstem levels.

LESION DATA IN SECTION 5

Many readers may consider the mapping of functions in Section 5 to be the key contribution of this atlas. If the assumption is correct that common deficits arising from focal lesions to different brain sites expose functional interrelationships among the brain sites involved, then Section 5 catalogs functional anatomies of a number of behavioral and physiological processes mediated within the brain of the rat. Some comments on these functional maps are in order.

1. Inspection of the 22 maps reveals that no single brain structure is solely involved in the expression of any given behavioral or physiological response. This finding may be considered to support the position (which falls somewhere between strict localization and strict nonlocalization) that functions, rather than being localized to a circumscribed ganglionic area or "center," depend on the combined activities of a constellation of nuclear groups whose elements may be widely dispersed throughout the neuraxis (Luria, 1966).

2. The finding that a number of different brain areas are essential for the normal expression of a given behavioral or physiological response helps to explain, at least in part, the almost ubiquitous recovery of function after brain damage (see Stein, Rosen, & Butters, 1974). Although several different explanations have been offered (Rosner, 1974), a likely one is that functional recovery results from incomplete destruction of those neural structures that are concerned with the execution of a particular response. A lucid account of this position has been presented by LeVere (1975).

3. As shown in Table 6-4, certain responses are more susceptible to interference by brain damage than are others. Changes in activity level on the observation table was the most commonly expressed deficit—of the 50 brain sites where lesions were placed, 40 were associated with either hyperkinesia or hypokinesia. Disturbances in the performance of previously learned responses were also frequently observed. It is instructive to note that the active avoidance and maze habits exhibited the lowest degree of localization within the brain (at least 35 of the 50 different lesion placements led to disruption of these learned responses), while the visual discrimination task was among the two habits exhibiting the highest degree of localization (only 21 of the 50 lesion placements led to disruption of this learned response). Interestingly, those investigators who have tended to view the neural circuitry of learning as involving diffuse networks of neurons occupying widespread regions of the brain have emphasized lesion research on the active avoidance and maze habits (John, 1972; Lashley, 1950). On the other hand, lesion research on visual discrimination tasks has been emphasized by those who tend to view the neural substrates of learning as involving relatively discrete pathways connecting one specific sector of the brain with another (Geshwind, 1965; Horel & Misantone, 1976; Mishkin, 1966; Myers, 1967; Thompson, 1965).

4. Among the deficits that appeared least frequently in the presence of brain damage were hyperphagia, somnolence, and coma (see Table 6-4). With respect to hyperphagia, it is likely that the use of a more sensitive measure of overeating (e.g.,

Table 6–3. Lesion-induced deficits in rats and humans: some similarities

| Rats | | Humans | | |
Deficit	Site of lesion	Deficit	Site of lesion	Reference
Visual discrimination	Occipito-temporal cortex	Blindness	Occipital lobe	Gloning et al., 1968
Maze	Parietal cortex	Route-walking	Parietal Lobe	Semmes et al., 1955
	Hippocampus	Stylus maze	Hippocampus	Milner et al., 1968
	Subthalamus	Porteus maze	Right subthalamus	Meier & Story, 1967
	Nigro-striate complex	Route-walking	Nigro-striate complex	Bowen et al., 1972
Aphagia-adipsia	Caudal medial forebrain bundle	Emaciation	Hypothalamus	Bauer, 1954
Hyperphagia	Ventromedial hypothalamus	Hyperphagia	Ventromedial hypothalamus	Reeves & Plum, 1969
Aggressiveness	Septal area	Physical assaultiveness	Septo-fornix area	Zeman & King, 1958
	Ventromedial hypothalamus	Rage	Ventromedial hypothalamus	Reeves & Plum, 1969
Abnormality of gait	Cerebellum	Locomotor ataxia	Cerebellum	Sypert & Alvord, 1975
Somnolence	Caudal medial forebrain bundle	Somnolence	Lateral hypothalamus	Sano et al., 1970
Coma	Midbrain central gray area	Coma	Central gray and adjacent tegmentum	Ingvar & Sourander, 1970
Defective pupilloconstrictor reflex	Pretectal area	Defective pupilloconstrictor reflex	Pretectal area	Christoff, 1974

food intake) than the one used in the current study would have disclosed more than three brain sites associated with this deficit. The investigation of the effects of smaller lesions might also have led to the identification of a greater number of brain sites associated with hyperphagia. Fonberg (1971; 1973), for example, has shown that small amygdaloid lesions may produce hyperphagia, while larger amygdaloid lesions may have no such effect.

Somnolence may also be associated with a greater number of brain sites than those indicated in Figure 5-18. Somnolence appeared in some animals sustaining either ventromedial thalamic or globus pallidus lesions, but the number of rats showing this disorder did not exceed 20% of the cases examined within each group. Conceivably, larger lesions placed within these areas may have disclosed a higher frequency of somnolence.

Coma was perhaps the most dramatic lesion-induced behavioral deficit observed in this study. It may be the most localized deficit studied as well. As shown in Figure 5-19, coma was observed in 25–49% of the cases having lesions in and around the mesencephalic central gray matter. Coma was not observed in any other brain-damaged rats of this study, except one: that rat had a lesion of the lateral lemniscal area with encroachment upon the central gray. It is important to note, however, that the mesencephalic focus for this deficit lies in an area immediately ventrolateral to the central gray. Coma was observed in 10 of 12 rats having Type II lesions to this area. The stereotaxic coordinates used to guide the lesion electrodes in these 12 rats were −0.5 mm frontal, 1.0 mm lateral, and 5.5 mm ventral (see Fig. 4-14). Unfortunately, this area was not selected for study in the construction of the behavioral atlas.

5. The illustrations presented in Section 5 disclose that no unique deficits arise from lesions to the neocortex. Any given deficit occurring with frontal, parietal, or occipito-temporal ablations was reproducible, at least in part, with discrete sub-

Table 6–4. The number of brain sites associated with a particular deficit

Deficit	Number of brain sites
Active avoidance	37
Maze	35
Vestibulo-kinesthetic discrimination	30
Escape response	28
Hyperkinesia	25
Aphagia-adipsia	22
Visual discrimination	21
Card displacement	20
Hypersensitivity	17
Hypokinesia	15
Aggressiveness	14
Defective labyrinthine reflex	12
Abnormality of gait	11
Obstinate progression	9
Hyperextension of the head	6
High mortality rate	5
Hypermetamorphosis	5
Jerky head movements	4
Defective pupilloconstrictor reflex	4
Coma	3
Hyperphagia	3
Somnolence	2

cortical lesions. These findings underscore the importance of subcortico-cortical and cortico-subcortical interactions in behavior and provide striking support for the argument that functions are organized on a vertical basis within the central nervous system, a notion advanced before the turn of the century by J. Hughlings Jackson (1890).

6. The first six maps of behavioral deficits shown in Section 5 deal with areas of the brain involved in the expression of previously learned responses. Examination of these maps reveals that certain areas are not centrally important for any of the learned responses (e.g., lateral lemniscal area); other areas are centrally important for all six learned responses (e.g., globus pallidus); and still other areas are centrally important for some learned responses, but not for others (e.g., parietal cortex). Although these findings bear upon many issues related to brain mechanisms and learning (see Thompson, Arabie & Sisk, 1976), only two will be considered briefly here; these will be considered in relation to Lashley's (1950) famous and still influential paper entitled "In Search of the Engram." The first issue revolves around the question of whether the entire cerebral cortex or a limited cortical region is essential for the performance of a learned activity. Lashley was inclined to favor the former view. However, it is apparent from the findings represented in the first six maps that each region of the cerebral cortex is not equipotential for the performance of any particular learned response: different habits depend on different cortical regions for their preservation. (Similar findings have come from ablation studies on the monkey—see Iverson, 1973.) The second issue revolves around the question of whether primacy should be attributed to the cerebral cortex alone or to the cerebral cortex in conjunction with subcortical formations in relation to learning and memory. Lashley was disposed to the view that the neocortex is the dominant level of the nervous system when it comes to learning and memory. However, inspection of the six maps reveals the importance of subcortical regions in the execution of every learned activity investigated in this study. In fact, comparisons of different brain regions in relation to cognitive complexity (see Table 6-2) suggest that the basal ganglia and the brainstem reticular formation may be more centrally involved in learning and memory than is the neocortex. These data together with the findings that decorticate animals can learn instrumental responses under unrestrained, free-moving conditions (Bjursten, Norrsell, & Norrsell, 1976; Oakley, 1971; Thompson, 1959) suggest that it may be necessary to reject the view that cortical processes take precedence over subcortical processes in the performance of any learned activity.

SUGGESTED READINGS

For those students who wish to pursue the psychobiology of the behavioral and physiological responses investigated in this atlas, some suggested sources of information are listed below.

Visual Discrimination Deficit
Isaacson, R. L. Experimental brain lesions and memory. In M. R. Rosenzweig & E. L. Bennett (Eds.), *Neural Mechanisms of Learning and Memory.* Cambridge: MIT Press, 1976, 521–543.
Thompson, R. Stereotaxic mapping of brainstem areas critical for memory of visual discrimination habits in the rat. *Physiological Psychology,* 1976, 4, 1–10.

Vestibulo-kinesthetic Discrimination Deficit
Thompson, R., Arabie, G. J. & Sisk, G. B. Localization of the "incline plane discrimination memory system" in the white rat. *Physiological Psychology,* 1976, 4, 311–324.

Card Displacement Deficit
Thompson, R. Card displacement response as affected by neocortical, cerebellar, and limbic forebrain lesions in the rat. *Bulletin of the Psychonomic Society,* 1976, 8, 101–102.
Thompson, R. Card displacement response as affected by brainstem lesions in the rat. *Bulletin of the Psychonomic Society,* 1976, 8, 103–104.

Maze Deficit
Lashley, K. S. *Brain Mechanisms and Intelligence.* Chicago: University of Chicago Press, 1929.
Thompson, R. Localization of the "maze memory system" in the white rat. *Physiological Psychology,* 1974, 2, 1–17.

Active Avoidance Deficit
Thomas, G. J., Hostetter, G. & Barker, D. J. Behavioral functions of the limbic system. In E. Stellar & J. M. Sprague (Eds.), *Progress in Physiological Psychology.* New York: Academic Press, 1968, Vol. 2, 230–311.
Vanderwolf, C. H. Limbic-diencephalic mechanisms of voluntary movement. *Psychological Review,* 1971, 78, 83–113.

Escape Response Deficit
Kirkby, R. J. & Kimble, D. P. Avoidance and escape behavior following striatal lesions in the rat. *Experimental Neurology,* 1968, 20, 215–227.

Liebman, J. M., Mayer, D. J. & Liebeskind, J. C. Mesencephalic central gray lesions and fear-motivated behavior in rats. *Brain Research,* 1970, 23, 353–370.
Stokes, L. D. & Thompson, R. Combined damage to the medial cerebral peduncle and anterior hypothalamus and escape behavior in the rat. *Journal of Comparative and Physiological Psychology,* 1970, 71, 303–310.

Hypermetamorphosis
Horel, J. A., Keating, E. G. & Misantone, L. J. Partial Klüver-Bucy syndrome produced by destroying temporal neocortex or amygdala. *Brain Research,* 1975, 94, 347–359.
White, N. & Weingarten, H. Effects of amygdaloid lesions on exploration by rats. *Physiology and Behavior,* 1976, 17, 73–79.

Obstinate Progression
Bailey, P. & Davis, E. W. The syndrome of obstinate progression in the cat. *Proceedings from the Society for Experimental Biology and Medicine,* 1942, 51, 307.

Hypokinesia
Hicks, L. H. & Birren, J. E. Aging, brain damage, and psychomotor slowing. *Psychological Bulletin,* 1970, 74, 377–396.
Thompson, R. & LeDoux, J. E. A stereotaxic map of brainstem areas critical for locomotor responses in a novel environment. *Bulletin of the Psychonomic Society,* 1975, 6, 327–328.

Hyperkinesia
Capobianco, S. & Hamilton, L. W. Effects of interruption of limbic system pathways on different measures of activity. *Physiology and Behavior,* 1976, 17, 65–72.

Hypersensitivity
Albert, D. J. & Richmond, S. E. Neural pathways mediating septal hyperreactivity. *Physiology and Behavior,* 1976, 17, 451–455.

Aphagia-adipsia and Hyperphagia
Grossman, S. P. Role of the hypothalamus in the regulation of food and water intake. *Psychological Review,* 1975, 82, 200–224.

Aggressiveness
Moyer, K. E. *The Psychobiology of Aggression.* New York: Harper & Row, 1976.

Jerky Head Movements
Marsden, C. D., Duvoisin, R. C., Jenner, P., Parkes, J. D., Pycock, C. & Tarsy, D. Relationship between animal models and clinical Parkinsonism. In D. Calne, T. N. Chase & A. Barbeau (Eds.), *Advances in Neurology.* New York: Raven Press, 1975, Vol. 9, 165–175.

Hyperextension of the Head
Pasik, P., Pasik, T. & Bender, M. B. The pretectal syndrome in monkeys: I. Disturbances of gaze and body posture. *Brain,* 1969, 92, 521–534.

Abnormality of Gait
Woodburne, L. S. Partial analysis of the neural elements in posture and locomotion. *Psychological Bulletin,* 1967, 68, 121–131.

Somnolence
Robinson, T. E. & Whishaw, I. Q. Effects of posterior hypothalamic lesions on voluntary behavior and hippocampal electroencephalograms in the rat. *Journal of Comparative and Physiological Psychology,* 1974, 86, 768–786.

Coma
Jefferson, G. The reticular formation and clinical neurology. In H. H. Jasper (Ed.), *Reticular Formation of the Brain.* Boston: Little, Brown, 1958, 729–738.

Defective Pupilloconstrictor Reflex
Legg, C. R. Effects of subcortical lesions on the pupillary light reflex in the rat. *Neuropsychologia,* 1975, 13, 373–376.

Defective Labyrinthine Reflex
Portegal, M., Abraham, L., Gilman, S. & Copack, P. Technique for vestibular neurotomy in the rat. *Physiology and Behavior,* 1975, 14, 217–221.
Thompson, R., Arabie, G. J. & Sisk, G. B. Localization of the "incline plane discrimination memory system" in the white rat. *Physiological Psychology,* 1976, 4, 311–324.

High Mortality Rate
Lanier, L. P., Petit, T. L., & Zornetzer, S. F. Discrete anterior medial thalamic lesions in the mouse: the production of acute postoperative hyperactivity and death. *Brain Research,* 1975, 91, 133–139.

BIBLIOGRAPHY

Bauer, H. D. Endocrine and other clinical manifestations of hypothalamic disease. *Journal of Clinical Endocrinology,* 1954, 14, 13–31.

Berntson, G. G. & Micco, D. J. Organization of brainstem behavioral systems. *Brain Research Bulletin,* 1976, 1, 471–483.

Bjursten, L. M., Norrsell, K. & Norrsell, U. Behavioral repertory of cats without cerebral cortex from infancy. *Experimental Brain Research,* 1976, 25, 115–130.

Bowen, F. P., Hoehn, M. M. & Yahr, M. D. Parkinsonism: Alterations in spatial orientation as determined by a route-walking test. *Neuropsychologia,* 1972, 10, 355–361.

Christoff, N. A clinicopathologic study of vertical eye movements. *Archives of Neurology,* 1974, 31, 1–8.

Fonberg, E. Hyperphagia produced by lateral amygdalar lesions in dogs. *Acta Neurobiologiae Experimentalis,* 1971, 31, 19–32.

Fonberg, E. The normalizing effect of lateral amygdalar lesions upon the dorsomedial amygdalar syndrome in dogs. *Acta Neurobiologiae Experimentalis,* 1973, 33, 449–466.

Gastaut, H. The role of the reticular formation in establishing conditioned reactions. In H. H. Jasper (Ed.), *Reticular formation of the brain.* Boston: Little, Brown, 1958, 561–579.

Geshwind, N. Disconnexion syndromes in animals and man. *Brain,* 1965, 88, 237–294.

Gloning, I. K., Gloning, K. & Hoff, H. *Neuropsychological symptoms and syndromes in lesions of the occipital lobe.* Paris: Gauthier-Villars, 1968.

Hart, B. L. *Experimental psychobiology.* San Francisco: W. H. Freeman, 1976.

Horel, J. A. & Misantone, L. J. Visual discrimination impaired by cutting temporal lobe connections. *Science,* 1976, 193, 336–338.

Ingvar, D. H. & Sourander, P. Destruction of the reticular core of the brain stem. *Archives of Neurology,* 1970, 23, 1–8.

Isaacson, R. L. Hippocampal destruction in man and other animals. *Neuropsychologia,* 1972, 10, 47–64.

Isaacson, R. L. Experimental brain lesions and memory. In M. R. Rosenzweig & E. L. Bennett (Eds.), *Neural mechanisms of learning and memory.* Cambridge: MIT Press, 1976, 521–543.

Iversen, S. D. Brain lesions and memory in animals. In J. A. Deutsch (Ed.), *The physiological basis of memory.* New York: Academic Press, 1973, 305–364.

Jackson, J. H. The Lumleian lectures on convulsive seizures. *British Medical Journal,* 1890, 1; 703–707, 765–771, 821–827.

John, E. R. Switchboard versus statistical theories of learning and memory. *Science,* 1972, 177, 850–864.

Klüver, H. & Bucy, P. C. Preliminary analysis of functions of the temporal lobes in monkeys. *Archives of Neurology and Psychiatry,* 1939, 42, 979–1000.

König, J. F. R. & Klippel, R. A. *The rat brain.* Baltimore: Williams & Wilkins, 1963.

Kornhuber, H. H. Cerebral cortex, cerebellum, and basal ganglia: An introduction to their motor functions. In F. O. Schmitt & F. G. Warden (Eds.), *The neurosciences. Third study program.* Cambridge: MIT Press, 1974, 267–280.

Krieg, W. J. S. Connections of the cerebral cortex: I. The albino rat: A. Topography of the cortical areas. *Journal of Comparative Neurology,* 1946, 84, 221–275.

Lashley, K. S. In search of the engram. *Symposia of the Society for Experimental Biology,* 1950, No. IV, 454–482.

Leonard, C. M. The prefrontal cortex of the rat. I. Cortical projections of the mediodorsal nucleus. II. Efferent connections. *Brain Research,* 1969, 12, 321–343.

LeVere, T. E. Neural stability, sparing, and behavioral recovery following brain damage. *Psychological Review,* 1975, 82, 344–358.

Luria, A. R. *Higher cortical functions in man.* New York: Basic Books, 1966.

Luria, A. R. The functional organization of the brain. *Scientific American,* 1970, 222, 66–78.

Lynch, G. Some difficulties associated with the use of lesion techniques in the study of memory. In M. R. Rosenzweig & E. L. Bennett (Eds.), *Neural mechanisms of learning and memory.* Cambridge: MIT Press, 1976, 544–546.

Maatsch, J. L. Learning and fixation after a single shock trial. *Journal of Comparative and Physiological Psychology,* 1959, 52, 408–410.

Mann, H. B. & Whitney, D. R. On a test of whether one or two random variables is stochastically larger than the other. *Annals of Mathematical Statistics,* 1947, 18, 50–60.

Marshall, J. F. & Teitelbaum, P. Further analysis of sensory inattention following lateral hypothalamic damage in rats. *Journal of Comparative and Physiological Psychology,* 1974, 84, 375–395.

Massopust, L. C. Stereotaxic atlases: A. Diencephalon of the rat. In D. E. Sheer (Ed.), *Electrical stimulation of the brain.* Austin: University of Texas Press, 1961, 182–202.

Meier, M. J. & Story, J. L. Selective impairment of Porteus maze test performance after right subthalamotony. *Neuropsychologia,* 1967, 5, 181–189.

Meyer, P. M. & Meyer, D. R. Neurosurgical procedures with reference to aspiration lesions. In R. D. Myers (Ed.), *Methods in psychobiology.* Vol. I, New York: Academic Press, 1971, 92–130.

Milner, B., Corkin, S. & Teuber, H.-L. Further analysis of the hippocampal amnestic syndrome: 14-year follow-up study of H. M. *Neuropsychologia,* 1968, 6, 215–234.

Mishkin, M. Visual mechanisms beyond the striate cortex. In R. W. Russell (Ed.), *Frontiers in physiological psychology.* New York: Academic Press, 1966, 93–119.

Moore, R. Y. & Heller, A. Monoamine levels and neuronal degeneration in rat brain following lateral hypothalamic lesions. *Journal of Pharmacology and Experimental Therapeutics,* 1967, 156, 12–22.

Myers, R. E. Cerebral connectionism and brain function. In C. H. Millikan & F. L. Darley (Eds.), *Brain mechanisms underlying speech and language.* New York: Grune and Stratton, 1967, 61–72.

Oakley, D. A. Instrumental learning in neodecorticate rabbits. *Nature (New Biology),* 1971, 233, 185–187.

Pellegrino, L. J. & Cushman, A. J. *A stereotaxic atlas of the rat brain.* New York: Appleton-Century-Crofts, 1967.

Penfield, W. & Mathieson, G. Memory. *Archives of Neurology,* 1974, 31, 145–154.

Pereboom, A. C. Some fundamental problems in experimental psychology: An overview. *Psychological Reports,* 1971, 28, 439–455.

Ploog, D. Vocal behavior and its "localization" as a prerequisite for speech. In K. J. Zülch, O. Creutzfeldt & G. C. Galbraith (Eds.), *Cerebral localization.* New York: Springer-Verlag, 1975, 229–236.

Reeves, A. G. & Plum, F. Hyperphagia, rage, and dementia accompanying a ventromedial hypothalamic neoplasm. *Archives of Neurology,* 1969, 20, 616–624.

Rosner, B. S. Recovery of function and localization of function in historical perspective. In. D. G. Stein, J. J. Rosen & N. Butters (Eds.), *Plasticity and recovery of function in the central nervous system.* New York: Academic Press, 1974, 1–29.

Sano, K., Mayanagi, Y., Sekino, H., Ogashiwa, M. & Ishejima, B. Results of stimulation and destruction of the posterior hypothalamus in man. *Journal of Neurosurgery,* 1970, 33, 689–707.

Sarnat, H. B. & Netsky, M. G. *Evolution of the nervous system.* New York: Oxford University Press, 1974.

Semmes, J., Weinstein, S., Ghent, L. & Teuber, H.-L. Spatial orientation in man after cerebral injury. I. Analysis by locus of lesion. *Journal of Psychology,* 1955, 39, 227–244.

Singh, D. & Avery, D. D. *Physiological techniques in behavioral research.* Monterey: Brooks-Cole, 1975.

Skinner, J. E. *Neuroscience: A laboratory manual.* Philadelphia: W. B. Saunders, 1971.

Stein, D. G., Rosen, J. J., & Butters, N. *Plasticity and recovery of function in the central nervous system.* New York: Academic Press, 1974.

Stellar, E. The physiology of motivation. *Psychological Review,* 1954, 61, 5–22.

Sypert, G. W. & Alvord, E. C. Cerebellar infarction. *Archives of Neurology,* 1975, 32, 357–363.

Thompson, R. Learning in rats with extensive neocortical damage. *Science,* 1959, 129, 1223–1224.

Thompson, R. Centrencephalic theory and interhemispheric transfer of visual habits. *Psychological Review,* 1965, 72, 385–398.

Thompson, R. Introducing subcortical lesions by electrolytic methods. In R. D. Myers (Eds.), *Methods in psychobiology.* Vol. I, New York: Academic Press, 1971, 131–154.

Thompson, R. Localization of the "maze memory system" in the white rat. *Physiological Psychology,* 1974, 2, 1–17.

Thompson, R., Arabie, G. J. & Sisk, G. B. Localization of the "incline plane discrimination memory system" in the white rat. *Physiological Psychology,* 1976, 4, 311–324.

Thompson, R. & Bryant, J. H. Memory as affected by activity of the relevant receptor. *Psychological Reports,* 1955, 1, 393–400.

Thompson, R., Duke., R. B., Malin, C. F. & Hawkins, W. F. The interpeduncular nucleus and retention in albino rats. *Journal of Comparative and Physiological Psychology,* 1961, 54, 329–333.

Ungerstedt, U. Adipsia and aphagia after 6-hydroxy-dopamine-induced degeneration of the nigrostriatal dopamine system. *Acta Physiologica Scandinavica,* 1971, Supplementum 367, 95–122.

Webster, W. G. Assumptions, conceptualizations, and the search for functions of the brain. *Physiological Psychology,* 1973, 1, 346–350.

Webster, W. G. *Principles of research methodology in physiological psychology.* New York: Harper & Row, 1975.

Young, R. M. *Mind, brain, and adaptation in the nineteenth century.* Oxford: Clarendon Press, 1970.

Zeigler, H. P. & Karten, H. J. Central trigeminal structures and the lateral hypothalamic syndrome in the rat. *Science,* 1974, 186, 636–638.

Zeman, W. & King, F. A. Tumors of the septum pellucidum and adjacent structures with abnormal affective behavior: An anterior midline structure syndrome. *Journal of Nervous and Mental Diseases,* 1958, 127, 490–502.

Zülch, K. J., Creutzfeldt, O. & Galbraith, G. C. *Cerebral localization.* New York: Springer-Verlag, 1975.

INDEX

Boldface page numbers refer to illustrations or maps.
Lesions and corresponding illustrations are listed on page 13; deficits
and corresponding maps, page 46.